Care of Children and Young People

RCGP Curriculum for
General Practice Series

Care of Children and Young People

A textbook for the nMRCGP

Edited by
Kay Mohanna

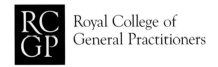

Royal College of
General Practitioners

The Royal College of General
Practitioners was founded in
1952 with this object:

*'To encourage, foster and maintain the
highest possible standards in general
practice and for that purpose to take or
join with others in taking steps consistent
with the charitable nature of that object
which may assist towards the same.'*

Among its responsibilities under
its Royal Charter the College is
entitled to:

*'Diffuse information on all matters
affecting general practice and issue
such publications as may assist the
object of the College.'*

British Library Cataloguing-in-Publication Data
A catalogue record for this book is available from
the British Library

© Royal College of General Practitioners 2009
Published by the Royal College of General
Practitioners 2009
14 Princes Gate, Hyde Park, London SW7 1PU

Disclaimer
This publication is intended for the use of medical
practitioners in the UK and not for patients. The
authors, editors and publisher have taken care to
ensure that the information contained in this book
is correct to the best of their knowledge, at the time
of publication. Whilst efforts have been made to
ensure the accuracy of the information presented,
particularly that related to the prescription of drugs,
the authors, editors and publisher cannot accept
liability for information that is subsequently shown
to be wrong. Readers are advised to check that the
information, especially that related to drug usage,
complies with information contained in the *British
National Formulary*, or equivalent, or manufacturers'
datasheets, and that it complies with the latest
legislation and standards of practice.

Designed and typeset at the Typographic Design Unit
Printed by Hobbs the Printers Ltd
Indexed by Carol Ball

ISBN: 978-0-85084-326-2

Contents

Contributors

Editor

Kay Mohanna is Senior Lecturer at Keele University School of Medicine and Director of Postgraduate Programmes. She is Chair of the Midland Faculty of the Royal College of General Practitioners and sits on the Central RCGP Council and the Postgraduate School of General Practice at the West Midlands Strategic Health Authority. Before entering general practice she worked in community paediatrics. Her research interests have included risk communication and informed consent, particularly with respect to research in pregnant women, and she has written extensively in medical education. She has three children, one of whom she sat up at nights with as a baby with asthma and who now plays centre for the school rugby first 15 – a triumph of determination over expectation in child health.

Contributing authors

Tony Choules studied Astronomy and Physics at University College London before training at University of Southampton Medical School. He graduated in Medicine in 1989 and trained in paediatrics in various hospitals across the south of England. He also trained for a year in Perth, Australia, before becoming a consultant paediatrician at Queen's Hospital, Burton upon Trent, in 1999. As well as his general paediatric work he has an interest in medical education and holds a Postgraduate Diploma in Medical Education. He is a Resuscitation Council UK instructor and course director. He is also College Tutor for Paediatrics and was recently appointed Postgraduate Clinical Tutor for Queen's Hospital.

Ilana Crome is Professor of Addiction Psychiatry at Keele University. She is also former Chair (1998–2002) of the Faculty of Substance Misuse at the Royal College of Psychiatrists, as well as a member of the Advisory Council on the Misuse of Drugs (ACMD) and the Executive Council of the Society for the Study of Addiction. She is Chair of an ACMD working group on treatment effectiveness. Her major clinical interest revolves around the development of innovative multidisciplinary, multi-agency services for young substance misusers. Her research activities include outcome research in young people, psychosocial risks, implementation and evaluation of multi-disciplinary training and education, and evidence-based policy responses to substance misuse problems.

Anthony Harnden is a GP in Wheatley, a Senior Lecturer at the Department of Primary Health Care at the University of Oxford and a Governing Body Fellow of St Hugh's College. His clinical and research interests are in primary care paediatrics, specifically common childhood infection, vaccine-preventable infection and the early diagnosis of serious disease. He has published a number of original articles, editorials and reviews in the topic area. He is the GP member of the Joint Committee of Vaccination and Immunisation and a board trustee of the Confidential Enquiry into Maternal and Child Health. He is the father of three teenagers.

Vince Ion has a wide range of experience in the public and private sectors including health care, education, and leadership within clinical settings. He is a qualified health visitor and nurse, and owns a consultancy business that focuses on his expertise in national policy development, modernisation in primary care, organisational change, widening participation, new role development, learning, mentoring and coaching. A life-changing family bereavement left him a single parent with two young children, causing him to leave his previous job as a marketing and sales director, and to train as a nurse and then a health visitor.

Andrew Mowat is a GP in rural Lincolnshire, where he is a GP educator. He is Child Health Lead for the RCGP and Chairman of the Primary Care Child Safeguarding Forum. He became involved in child protection after realising the positive difference that support of a GP can make to the outcome for a child in need. Since 1999 he has chaired his practice's multi-agency child protection team, and has been the named doctor for child protection for the East Lincolnshire Primary Care Trust. He is married with two children, and is actively involved with the British Medical Association, as Honorary Secretary of the Lincoln Division and Chairman of the Conference of Honorary Secretaries of BMA Divisions. When not protecting the rights of children or doctors, he sings with the Partney Choir, a small community and church choir in rural East Lincolnshire.

Moli Paul is an Associate Clinical Professor at the University of Warwick and an honorary consultant child and adolescent psychiatrist within a multi-disciplinary Child and Adolescent Mental Health Service in South Warwickshire. Having graduated from the University of Birmingham Medical

School, Moli worked as a junior doctor in a number of specialities, including paediatrics and neonatology, before completing her postgraduate training in Psychiatry in the West Midlands. She has a PhD in Biomedical Ethics and teaches undergraduates and postgraduates on communicating with children and young people, child and adolescent psychiatry, and ethics. Her research interests include healthcare decision-making by children, young people and their families, empirical research on consent and rights, health services research (including transitions between adolescent and adult health services), user involvement and the sociology of childhood and adolescence, and how it affects healthcare provision and utilisation.

Mohammad Sawal is a Consultant Paediatrician. He is Lead in Neurology and Neurodisability at Queen's Hospital, Burton upon Trent, and South Staffordshire Foundation Trust. His paediatric training was in the West Midlands and he is a mentor at the University of Birmingham Medical School. His research interests are children with visual impairments, epilepsy and neurodisability. His wife is a GP and they have two children.

Matthew Thompson is a GP and Clinical Lecturer in Primary Health Care based at the University of Oxford's Department of Primary Health Care. He received his medical degree from the University of Glasgow, and has combined GP training and living in both the UK and the USA. He holds an MPH from the University of Washington and a DPhil from the University of Oxford. He spent a year working as a rural doctor in KwaZulu, South Africa, and worked in the USA for 8 years. He has taught medical students and GP trainees on primary care and evidence-based medicine. His research interests include educational needs assessment, health workforce studies, and more recently primary research on various paediatric health topics in general practice. Currently he is co-ordinating research looking at better ways of identifying children with serious illness in primary care, and using new diagnostic technologies in primary care.

Joyce Williams grew up in the West Midlands and studied Medicine at the University of Birmingham. She trained on the Black Country Vocational Training Scheme and has worked as a GP in the West Midlands since then. She has been involved in working parties for setting up and updating child health surveillance/child health promotion programmes in the West Midlands and has worked in family planning for the past 12 years. She has an MSc in Community Gynaecology and an MMedEd in Medical Education, both from the University of Warwick. She plays an active part in education of both GP registrars and medical students, and has also been involved in training in family planning since 2003. She became an MRCGP examiner in 2003 and is now involved in the nMRCGP as a CSA assessor and in CSA training courses for GP registrars.

Preface

In the week the finishing touches were being put to this book, the news was grim in the field of child protection. The case of Baby P, the 17-month-old boy who died in August 2007 after suffering sustained abuse and over 50 injuries, was once again focusing attention on the care given by health and social care professionals to vulnerable children. This case came to court just 6 months after Khyra Ishaq, aged 7, apparently starved to death in Birmingham in May 2008.

It seems the lessons in the Laming Report following the inquiry into the death of 8-year-old Victoria Climbié in 2000 have not been learned. The Climbié report and subsequent national audit of services for cases where neglect or abuse are suspected had highlighted the need for changes in the training and organisation of those working in child services. The priority areas were identified as: obtaining and recording relevant information about children; referral and communication between different agencies; carrying out prompt and effective assessment and investigations; and timely recording and auditing of decisions and actions.

These priority areas equally well apply to the general health care of children. Trainees entering general practice need to be able to demonstrate by the end of their training period that they have acquired the knowledge, skills and attitudes to be the advocate for children. The GP curriculum statement on the care of children and young people identifies the key areas for professional development. This book has been designed to support those in training and undergoing the new GP assessment process, and can also act as an update for established practitioners who have demonstrated learning needs in child and adolescent health in their appraisal and are preparing for revalidation.

The United Kingdom has one of the highest teenage pregnancy rates in Europe and growing problems with drug and alcohol addiction, childhood obesity and behavioural problems. Of course none of these can be addressed by GPs alone. One of the themes throughout this book is teamwork and communication with others including parents, health visitors and midwives, child and adolescent psychiatrists, social services, teachers, paediatricians and community paediatricians. The team of authors has been assembled to reflect this mix and we hope will in itself illustrate the benefits of working together to do the best for children.

Kay Mohanna
August 2009

Foreword

I am delighted to provide a foreword to this very useful book.

The health of children and young people is in the spotlight as never before. The delivery of health care is changing and their needs have not always been in the forefront of our minds in recent times. This is changing too.

Modern care for children requires a breadth and depth of knowledge skills and competencies, across the full range from newborn to young adult, from promotion of health and prevention of illness, through first contact with the acutely ill child and the management of long-term conditions or disabilities.

We must understand the importance of good parenting, the need to safeguard children and ensure we focus on the emotional aspects as well as the physical ones. Disability, adolescence and transition to adult services need a new approach too. Primary care is well placed to tackle these vital areas while ensuring optimal health for the next generation.

I welcome this book. I hope it will inspire those in training and their trainers to bring themselves up to date with modern evidence-based practice and help them develop the knowledge and confidence needed to work with children, young people and their families, which is so rewarding.

Dr Sheila Shribman
National Clinical Director
Children, Young People and Maternity Services
Department of Health, Partnerships for Children,
Family and Maternity Division
August 2009

Abbreviations

A&E	Accident and Emergency
AABR	automated auditory brainstem response
ADD	attention deficit disorder
ADH	antidiuretic hormone
ADHD	attention deficit hyperactivity disorder
AOM	acute otitis media
ASD	autistic spectrum disorder
AYPH	Association for Young People's Health
BMI	body mass index
BTS	British Thoracic Society
CAF	common assessment framework
CAMHS	Child and Adolescent Mental Health Services
CBT	cognitive behavioural therapy
CMPI	cow's milk protein intolerance
COCP	combined oral contraceptive pill
CONI	Care of the Next Infant
CSCS	Children's Social Care Services
DDH	developmental dysplasia of the hip
DLA	Disability Living Allowance
DVT	deep vein thrombosis
ENT	ear, nose and throat
EURACT	European Academy of Teachers in General Practice
GABA	gamma-aminobutyric acid
GMS	General Medical Services
GORD	gastro-oesophageal reflux disease
GPStR	general practice specialty registrar
GPwSI	GP with a special interest
GTCS	generalised tonic-clonic seizures
HBSC	Health Behaviour in School-Aged Children
HiB	*Haemophilus influenzae* type B
HPV	human papillomavirus
ISD	Information Services Division
IUCD	intrauterine contraceptive device
LABA	long-acting beta-2 agonists
LARCs	long-acting contraceptives
LRA	leukotriene receptor antagonist
MCADD	medium-chain acyl-CoA dehydrogenase deficiency
MMR	measles, mumps and rubella

NEETs	not in education, employment or training
NICE	National Institute for Health and Clinical Excellence
NNT	number needed to treat
NSF	National Service Framework
NSPCC	National Society for the Prevention of Cruelty to Children
OAE	oto-acoustic emission
PCT	primary care trust
PDDs	pervasive developmental disorders
PEFR	peak expiratory flow rate
PKU	phenylketonuria
pMDI	pressurised metered dose inhaler
PMS	Personal Medical Services
POP	progesterone-only pill
PR	parental responsibility
RCGP	Royal College of General Practitioners
RCP	Royal College of Physicians
SENCO	Special Educational Needs Co-ordinator
SID	Sudden Infant Death
SIGN	Scottish Intercollegiate Guidelines Network
STI	sexually transmitted infection
SUDEP	Sudden Unexpected Death in Epilepsy
TB	tuberculosis
UNICEF	United Nations Children's Fund
URTI	upper respiratory tract infections
UTI	urinary tract infection
WAVE	wheeze-associated viral episode
WHO	World Health Organization

How does our society care for children and young people?

Preconception to adulthood

Kay Mohanna

Introduction

A recent essay in the *British Journal of General Practice* notes that there are growing concerns about the health of children and young people in the UK.[1]

In the UK there are approximately:[2]

▷ 12 million children and young people aged 18 and younger
  (more than the entire population of many European countries)
▷ 6 million young people aged under 10
▷ 600,000 live births a year
▷ 1 million children with mental health disorders
▷ 400,000 children and young people in need
▷ 320,000 disabled children and young people
▷ 59,700 looked-after children and young people.

Their vulnerability, combined with their inability when young to articulate what they are feeling, poses a challenge for everyone involved in health and social care.

The United Nations Children's Fund (UNICEF) reported in 2007 on an overview of child wellbeing in rich countries, and found Britain came in last, trailing in twenty-first place.[3] The report collates replies on over 40 separate indicators in six groups: material wellbeing, health and safety, education, peer and family relationships, behaviours and risks, and subjective wellbeing. The UK is bottom of the table overall, and bottom for five of the six groups of indicators on such issues as high poverty, high infant mortality and low birthweight, poor family and peer relationships, high levels of alcohol use, early sexual activity and teenage pregnancy, high numbers of those aged 16–18 who are not in education, employment or training ('NEETs') and finally low self-assessed wellbeing.

Home Office figures from the 2003 report *Hidden Harm: responding to the needs of children of problem drug users* make alarming reading:[4]

▷ 300,000 children are estimated to live with a drug-misusing parent – representing about 2–3 per cent of children under 16
▷ 850,000 children live with a parent who misuses alcohol – this brings with it the potential consequences of social deprivation and the physical impact through foetal alcohol spectrum
▷ 30–50 per cent of adult mental health users are parents
▷ there are estimated to be 175,000 young carers in the UK, who have a high risk of mental health problems.

One response has been the formation of a new charity, the Association for Young People's Health (AYPH), and the Royal College of General Practitioners (RCGP) Adolescent Task Group is a main partner in that development.

Much of what is needed to address this is not directly in the health remit. The World Health Organization's (WHO) framework for programming for young people's health and development reflects this[5] and is reproduced in Table 1.1.

Table 1.1 ○ **Contribution of different professional sectors in programming for young people's health**

	Health sector	Education sector	Media	And many others: labour, criminal justice, social services, parents, peers, etc.
Information and life skills	+	+++	++	++
Services and counselling	+++	+	+	+
Safe and supportive environment	+	++	++	+++
Opportunities to participate	+	+	+	++

The WHO further expands that by listing the priorities for the health sector:

▷ collect, analyse and disseminate the data that are required for advocacy, policies and programmes
▷ provide services that include a focus on prevention, treatment and rehabilitation
▷ support the development of evidence-informed policies and strategies that provide vision and guidance
▷ mobilise, support and co-ordinate with other sectors.

There are thus policy and strategic responsibilities for governments, guided by health advisers including those in primary care.

The role of individual GPs in the care of children and adolescents at a local level is crucial. All GPs need to be trained in the care of children and young people. They should be able to treat them when sick, help them to keep healthy, prevent illness, respond effectively to child protection issues and help them and their parents to cope with chronic illness and disability. Crucially, GPs are generalists. This means they are skilled in managing illness in its early stages, balancing risks, dealing with uncertainty and then knowing when and to whom to refer. General practice specialty registrars (GPStRs) need an all-round training in child health issues; it is not a special interest.

The RCGP curriculum recognises the fundamental importance of this area of practice in statement 8 of the new GP curriculum. This can be found at www.rcgp-curriculum.org.uk/pdf/curr_8_Care_of_Children_and_Young_People.pdf.

This book seeks to be a key resource for GPStRs to increase the effectiveness of the services and care they provide to children and young people. It is based on and expands resources that are listed in the curriculum statement. To set the scene for future chapters, in this chapter we have reproduced some of the background published in that statement.

3

Early years

A child's experience in early life – and even before birth – has a crucial impact on his or her life chances. There is good evidence from Starfield in the USA that providing early-years care in the primary care setting delivers improved child health outcomes. Health indicators such as the percentage of infants born with low birthweight and post-neonatal mortality are better in countries with better developed primary care.[6-8]

Within the primary healthcare team prenatal care and healthy lifestyle advice to support parents is key. The role of fathers in contributing to their child's development and wellbeing is important, and their part in parenting their children should not be overlooked. Parents need information to help them make informed decisions about the needs of their children, and efforts should be made to ensure that consistent advice and information is given to parents across different care settings.

Useful information provided locally to parents might include:[9]

▷ what becoming a parent might be like and what it will involve
▷ the importance of pre-conceptual folic acid, and promoting health during pregnancy, not smoking during pregnancy and having a smoke-free atmosphere
▷ how to breastfeed and, where this is not possible, how to bottle-feed safely; healthy weaning at the appropriate age
▷ reducing the risks of sudden infant death, accident prevention, reducing non-intentional injury, first aid and basic life-saving skills for children
▷ the importance of parents communicating with their babies from birth
▷ how to nurture babies, children and young people, set appropriate boundaries and manage behaviour effectively
▷ healthy lifestyles, including skills and knowledge of the purchase and preparation of food to form a balanced diet, the importance of an active lifestyle and of maintaining a healthy weight
▷ what to expect at different ages, including emotional development, growth, puberty and child and adolescent development
▷ the importance of creating play opportunities for learning, how to create an effective learning environment at home from the early years, and how to engage effectively in a child's and young person's cognitive, emotional and social development
▷ common allergies and how to manage allergic reactions
▷ a range of other health issues, including emotional health and wellbeing, bullying, sex and relationships, and alcohol, tobacco and drug and substance misuse
▷ services to support parents, children and young people through disrupted relationships and bereavement
▷ how to promote and support independence as young people grow up
▷ how to access services for their children, how to discuss and/or respond to health and wellbeing issues
▷ the legal concept of 'parental responsibility', and information that explains the rights of both the parent and the child, and young people in the family.

Prenatal screening

Healthy childhoods begin with healthy pregnancies. Further information on this aspect can be found in RCGP curriculum statement 10.1 *Women's Health* and supporting resources.

The current prenatal screening policy for England is listed in Table 1.2. There is some variation in Scotland and Wales.

Table 1.2 ○ *Prenatal screening*

Anaemia	All pregnant women
Asymptomatic bacteriuria in pregnancy	All pregnant women
Blood group and RhD status, and atypical red-cell alloantibodies	All pregnant women
Down's syndrome	All pregnant women
Foetal anomalies including neural tube defects	All pregnant women
Hepatitis B	All pregnant women
HIV	All pregnant women
Psychiatric illness	Offered to those with psychiatric history to detect possible relapse early
Rubella immunity	All pregnant women
Sickle cell and thalassaemia	▶ Enhance lab screening for all women served by Primary Care Trusts with high prevalence areas (prevalence of sickle cell > 1.5/10,000 pregnancies) ▶ low prevalence (definition = foetal prevalence of sickle cell < 1.5/10,000 pregnancies) should offer screening using the recommended Family Origin Question as well as a formal process of inspection of routine blood indices to screen for thalassaemia
Syphilis	All pregnant women
Tay–Sachs disease	At-risk population (Ashkenazi Jewish people)

Newborn screening is listed in Table 1.3.

Table 1.3 ○ *Newborn screening*

Congenital hypothyroidism	All newborn babies
Cystic fibrosis	All newborn babies
Medium-chain acyl-CoA dehydrogenase deficiency (MCADD)	All newborn babies in England since May 2009
Phenylketonuria (PKU)	All newborn babies
Sickle cell and thalassaemia	All newborn babies in high-prevalence areas

Children aged 4 and under visit their GP on average six times a year, while school-age children and young people visit two or three times.[10] This means that contact with parents, and the opportunity to guide them and respond to their concerns, is high in primary care.

UK child health policy

Following a series of high-profile cases including the Laming report of the inquiry into the death of Victoria Climbié, who died in 2000, and the Kennedy report following the Bristol Heart Inquiry, the first Minister of State for Children at the Department for Education and Skills was appointed in 2003. She took responsibility for children's services, child care and provision for under-5s, as well as family policy (including parenting support and family law).

In September 2003, the government launched the green paper *Every Child Matters.*[11] It proposed a range of measures to reform and improve children's care and to protect children from neglect and harm. Later, in March 2004, *Every Child Matters: next steps*[12] was published on the same day as the Children Bill was introduced to parliament. This document set out the purpose of the Children Bill and the next steps for bringing about change of children's services.

In 2004, *The National Service Framework for Children, Young People and Maternity Services*[10] was published ('The Children's NSF'). This launched the new Child Health Promotion Programme, based in part on *Health for All Children.*[13]

The core Child Health Promotion Programme encompasses:

▷ childhood screening
▷ immunisations
▷ a holistic and systematic process to assess the needs of the individual child, young person and family

6

▷ early interventions to address those needs
▷ delivering universal health-promoting activities.

The Programme is:

▷ offered to all children and young people throughout childhood and the
teenage years in a range of settings
▷ delivered in general practices, children's centres, early-years providers
and extended schools
▷ provided as an additional service under the General Medical Services
(GMS) contract and through local Personal Medical Services (PMS)
contracts
▷ a universal service that is individualised to meet the needs of the child,
young person and family
▷ designed to support on a targeted basis children and families who are
vulnerable or have complex needs
▷ delivered in partnership with parents to help them make healthy
choices for their children, adolescents and family.

7

The year 2004 also saw the important issue of child poverty assessed with
Child Poverty Review,[14] a report from the Treasury that examined the welfare
reform and public service changes necessary to advance towards the long-
term goal of halving child poverty by 2010 and eradicating it by 2020. The
review set out the key measures to reduce child poverty in the medium to
long term, in particular through improving poor children's life chances. It
summarised continued efforts to help parents who want to return to work,
providing financial support to families and tackling material deprivation.

Later that year, a further ten modules of the Children's NSF were launched,
setting aspirations for the improvement of services across health, education
and social care for women, children and their families for the next 10 years.

In November 2004, the white paper on public health *Choosing Health:
making healthy choices easier* was published,[15] which set out the key principles
for supporting the public to make healthier and more informed choices in
regards to their health. Chapter 2, 'Children and young people: starting on
the right path', builds on earlier initiatives in child health.

The Children Act of 2004 provides a legislative spine for the wider strategy for improving children's lives. This covers the universal services that
every child accesses, and more targeted services for those with additional
needs. The overall aim is to encourage integrated planning, commissioning
and delivery of services, as well as to improve multidisciplinary working,
remove duplication, increase accountability and improve the co-ordination
of individual and joint inspections in local authorities.

The legislation is enabling rather than prescriptive and provides local authorities with a considerable amount of flexibility in the way they implement its provisions.

The Department for Education and Skills green paper *Youth Matters*[16] was published in 2005 and outlined a plan that encouraged joint working between health, social services and education when meeting the needs of young people. This was in an attempt to address the perceived risk that too many vulnerable young people were falling through gaps in service provision. In part this is seen as a result of the various divisions between services and a lack of communication and collaboration between them. This was not without controversy, some seeing it as an attack on the civil rights of young people by extending surveillance and control over them.[17]

In October 2005 the Department of Health published *You're Welcome quality criteria*,[18] developed from the *Getting it Right for Teenagers in Your Practice*[19] advanced by the Adolescent Task Group of the RCGP with the Royal College of Nursing.

Similar initiatives have been implemented in each of the devolved countries and up-to-date details can be found in RCGP curriculum statement 8 *Care of Children and Young People.*

Asset models to enhance the health of our children and young people

A lot of work has been done in recent years looking at those attributes of communities that can enhance the health of children and young people. For over two decades the WHO Child and Adolescent Health Research Unit has been looking at all such aspects in the Health Behaviour in School-Aged Children (HBSC) cross-national study, now covering 43 countries.[20] Anthony Morgan, principal investigator for the England site, states:[21]

Much of the evidence base available to address inequalities is based on a 'deficit model' of health. Deficit models focus on identifying problems and needs of populations requiring professional resources. This can result in high levels of dependence on hospital and welfare services.

In contrast asset models tend to accentuate positive ability, capability and capacity to identify problems and activate solutions, which promote the self esteem of individuals and communities leading to less reliance on professional services.

A health asset can be defined as any factor (or resource), which enhances the ability of individuals, communities and populations to maintain and sustain health and well-being.

These assets can operate at the level of the individual, family or community as protective (and/or promoting) factors to buffer against life's stresses.

The Minneapolis Search Institute has published work examining US communities for signs of such 'assets' that can promote and enhance the health of children and young people.[22] This work has identified 40 development assets that can be listed under seven groupings:

▷ **support** ▶ (family relationships, caring school and neighbourhood)
▷ **empowerment** ▶ (the community values young people, who are seen as resources)
▷ **constructive use of time** ▶ (participation in clubs and associations)
▷ **commitment to learning** ▶ (achievement, motivation)
▷ **positive values** ▶ (caring and responsible to others)
▷ **social competences** ▶ (cultural competence, peaceful conflict resolution)
▷ **positive identity** ▶ (self-esteem).

Our aim must be to develop capability and resilience in our youngsters. In general practice, with our longitudinal relationships with patients and their families, some of that should be possible.

So, with an understanding of the context within which we work, how has this been taken into account in developing the RCGP curriculum? What aspects do trainees (and practices) need to consider in order to become competent to look after children and their families (and stay up to date and maintain their fitness to practise in this area)?

The RCGP domains of competence: six core competences for GPs

The RCGP curriculum on *Care of Children and Young People* can be found in full on the RCGP website.[23] Like all the curriculum statements it is based on the WONCA definition of primary care and covers six core domains.[24]

The first three domains have as their focal point the primary care consultation. They are:

1 ▷ Primary care management
2 ▷ Person-centred care
3 ▷ Specific problem-solving skills.

The remaining domains are more complex and take a wider perspective, going beyond the consulting room GP–patient interaction:

4 ▷ A comprehensive approach

5 ▷ Community orientation

6 ▷ A holistic approach.

All six of these are 'rooted' in an understanding of the scientific basis, attitudinal and contextual aspects – known as the three essential features.

These core competences and characteristics have been drawn from the European Academy of Teachers in General Practice (EURACT) Educational Agenda and are represented in Figure 1.1.

What follows is a summary of these competences. It is important to consult the full document on the RCGP website.

Primary care management

This competence is about managing primary contact with children and their families, and recognises the importance of multi-agency working (working across professional and agency boundaries). The welfare of the child and young person must be the paramount consideration and can help to justify actions that challenge ethical and professional norms.

GPs must ensure that parents or carers, children and young people receive information, advice and support to enable them as much as possible to manage both minor and chronic illnesses themselves. It is important to take into account an understanding of the needs of ethnic minorities and cultural differences in beliefs about illness and the use of medicines.

Trainees must demonstrate an understanding of the welfare of the unborn baby by being aware of the impact of parental problems including domestic violence, substance misuse and mental health problems.

Person-centred care

GPs need to adopt a family-centred approach in dealing with patients, their families and their problems. This requires effective communication and engagement to enable parents or carers, children and young people to participate in their own care. It will be vital to understand the problems with transitions from child to adolescent, and from adolescent to adult, including managing the transition from one set of healthcare professionals in paediatrics, to those in adult medicine.

Specific problem-solving skills

Those involved in the care of children and young adults need to use a decision-making process determined by the prevalence and incidence of illness in the

Figure 1.1 ○ *WONCA tree of family medicine*

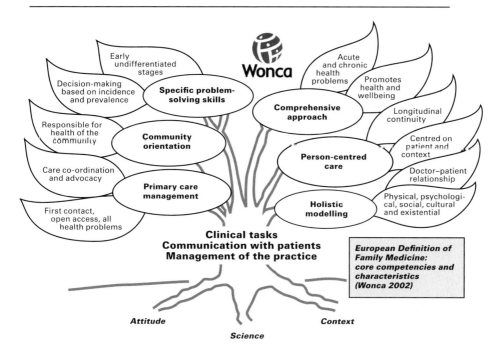

Source: ©2004 Swiss College of Primary Care Medicine. Used by permission.

community and the specific circumstances of the patient and family, being aware of normal growth and development of children and young people.

A comprehensive approach

Managing simultaneously both acute and chronic conditions in the same child is challenging and can be helped by assessing children and young people's developmental needs in the context of their family and environmental factors, such as school and community, as well as parenting capacity. It will be necessary to be familiar with the issues involved in delivering services for young people relating to access, communication, confidentiality and consent.

Community orientation

GPs reconcile the health needs of patients and their families, and of the community in which they live, in balance with available resources. This requires an understanding of the legal and political context of child and adolescent care, and an understanding of the organisation of care.

11

A holistic approach

It is important to support transitions in life stages to enable families to maximise their children's achievements and opportunities, and understand their rights and responsibilities. This is especially true when supporting those families living with a child with a disability or chronic disease.

Contextual aspects

The healthcare needs of the paediatric population are affected by the socio-economic and cultural features of the community. There are important workload issues raised by paediatric problems, especially the demand for urgent consultation and the mechanisms for dealing with this.

Attitudinal aspects

Children and young people must be treated equitably, and with respect for their beliefs, preferences, dignity and rights. Record-keeping and appropriate sharing of information are important.

Scientific aspects

In many ways the basis of healthcare provision for children and young people is exactly the same as for adults. GPs must access information on the best evidence about the effectiveness of interventions, weigh up and evaluate evidence, and consider whether research findings are applicable in each context. Significant events should be recorded and used in multidisciplinary and multi-agency audits.

Conclusion

There is much to be done in the provision of health care for children and young adults to address some of the challenges discussed in this chapter.

The role of the GP in the multidisciplinary team is key. As we have seen, GPs are generalists:

The generalist is a skilled diagnostician, working by pattern recognition, absorbing risks and uncertainty about patients' presenting problems but at the same time operating fail-safe processes to ensure patient safety. ... [The GP trainee] needs to develop the ability to see in over-view, filter and clarify and signpost patients to interventions either administered by them or other members of the primary care team or those in secondary care. They need broad clinical expertise but also additional values-based abilities to lead individualised discussions with patients.[25]

In subsequent chapters we will look more closely at what a GPStR needs to know to be able to do develop these skills and carry out this role effectively.

Acknowledgements

This chapter includes some material that was originally published in the RCGP curriculum statement 8. The work of Professor Yvonne Carter as statement guardian and the statement authors Dr Stephen Kelly, Dr Ruth Bastable, Dr Mike Deighan, Professor Steve Field and Dr Amar Rughani is acknowledged.

References

1 • Roberts J. Launch of the Association for Young People's Health *British Journal of General Practice* 2008; **58(551)**: 447.

2 • www.statistics.gov.uk/glance/#population [accessed August 2009].

3 • The United Nations Children's Fund. *Child Poverty in Perspective: an overview of child health in rich countries* Florence, Italy: UNICEF, 2007.

4 • Advisory Council on the Misuse of Drugs. *Hidden Harm: responding to the needs of children of problem drug users* London: Home Office, 2003.

5 • World Health Organization. *Child and Adolescent Health and Development: progress report 2006–2007* Geneva: WHO, 2007.

6 • Starfield B. Is primary care essential? *Lancet* 1994; **344**: 1129–33.

7 • Starfield B. *Primary Care, Health, and Equity Part I* (based on data in Starfield B, Shi L. Policy relevant determinants of health: an international perspective *Health Policy* 2002; **60(3)**: 201–18), www.pitt.edu/~super1/lecture/lec17361/011.htm [accessed August 2009].

8 • Starfield B. *Primary Care, Health, and Equity Part II: rates of avoidable hospitalizations for diabetes mellitus and pneumonia among children were lower in areas where the family physician to population ratios were higher, but this was not the case for the paediatrician to population ratio* (in Starfield B, Shi L. Policy relevant determinants of health: an international perspective *Health Policy* 2002; **60(3)**: 201–18).

9 • Department for Education and Skills. *Birth to Three Matters* London: DfES 2002, www.surestart.gov.uk [accessed August 2009].

10 • Department of Health. *National Service Framework for Children, Young People and Maternity Services* London: DoH, 2004.

11 • Department for Education and Skills. *Every Child Matters* London: DfES, 2003.

12 • Department for Education and Skills. *Every Child Matters: next steps* Nottingham: DfES, 2004, www.everychildmatters.gov.uk/_files/A39928055378AF27E9122D73 4BF10F74.pdf [accessed August 2009].

13 • Hall D, Elliman D. *Health for All Children* (4th edn) Oxford: Oxford University Press, 2003.

14 • HM Treasury. *Child Poverty Review* London: HM Treasury, 2004.

15 • Department of Health. *Choosing Health: making healthy choices easier* London: DoH, www.dh.gov.uk/en/Publicationsandstatistics/Publications/PublicationsPolicyAnd Guidance/DH_4094550 [accessed August 2009].

16 • Department for Education and Skills. *Youth Matters* London: DfES, 2005.

17 • Smith M K. *Youth Matters*: the green paper for youth 2005, *The Encyclopaedia of Informal Education*, 2005, www.infed.org/youthwork/green_paper_2005.htm [accessed August 2009].

18 • Department of Health. *You're Welcome Quality Criteria: making health services young people friendly* London: DoH, 2005.

19 • Royal College of General Practitioners, Royal College of Nursing. *Getting it Right for Teenagers in Your Practice* London: RCGP, 2002.

20 • Morgan A, Malam S, Muir J, *et al. Health and Social Inequalities in English Adolescents: exploring the importance of school, family and neighbourhood, findings from the WHO Health Behaviour in School-Aged Children Study* London: NICE, 2006.

21 • Bartley M (ed.) on behalf of the ESRC Priority Network on Capability and Resilience. *Capability and Resilience: beating the odds* London: UCL Department of Epidemiology and Public Health, 2006.

22 • Benson P. *All Kids are Our Kids: what communities must do to raise caring and responsible children and adolescents* San Francisco: Jossey-Bass, 2006.

23 • Royal College of General Practitioners. *Care of Children and Young People* (curriculum statement 8) London: RCGP, 2007, www.rcgp-curriculum.org.uk/pdf/curr_8_Care_of_ Children_and_Young_People.pdf [accessed August 2009].

24 • WONCA Europe. *The European Definition of General Practice/Family Medicine* London: WONCA Europe; 2005.

25 • Mohanna K, Tavabie A, Chambers R. The renaissance of generalism *Education for Primary Care* 2006; **17**: 425–31.

Care of the newborn

Joyce Williams

2

Introduction

When a baby is born an early question most parents ask is,

▷ *'Is my baby normal?'*

In primary care, it is the role of a number of healthcare professionals to screen the new baby for important medical conditions and for any sign of deviation from normal development. Examination and developmental assessment along with health promotion and advice is collectively known as the child health surveillance programme. Although it has always been the case that the family doctor is available for support and advice for young families as well as medical care, it was first formally introduced in the UK in 1989, following the publication of the white paper *Working for Patients*.[1] This chapter looks at the first few weeks of life and the role of the multidisciplinary primary care team during this period.

Child health surveillance

When child health surveillance was introduced in the UK it was funded under a new contract for GPs, to be delivered to all children under the age of five, by GPs who were registered on their local child health surveillance list. Registration was subject to discretionary decisions by local health authorities about GPs' eligibility. The parents received a hand-held child medical record (often referred to as 'the red book'), which included growth charts, screening examinations results, a place for comments that all healthcare professionals could access and general advice about developmental milestones, managing minor ailments, etc.

This programme continued for many years, with minor improvements and modifications, until the publication of the *National Service Framework for Children, Young People and Maternity Services* in 2004,[2] which launched the 'Child Health Promotion Programme'. This new programme includes:

▷ childhood screening

▷ holistic assessment of the needs of the child and family
▷ early interventions, when indicated
▷ promotion of health in children (including immunisations).

Examination of the newborn child

The examination of the newborn child and the 6-week check are similar examinations, both aimed at detecting medical problems and possibly some early signs of developmental problems.

The baby is carefully examined all over, looking for problems such as congenital abnormalities, asymmetry of body posture, and asymmetry of limb movements. Primitive reflexes are checked and the baby is systematically examined. A tick-box checklist is useful to ensure that nothing is missed out, an example of which is shown in Box 2.1.

Box 2.1 ○ *Early examination*

Appearance ▶ Does the baby look 'normal'? Is there anything unusual?

Nutrition ▶ Are the growth charts within normal or expected limits? Does the baby look over- or under-fed?

Fontanelles ▶ Are the fontanelles of normal size and number? Is the tension normal?

Palate ▶ Is there an underlying bony cleft?

Eyes ▶ Is the 'red reflex' present? Do the eyes 'follow'? Is there evidence of a squint?

Hearing ▶ Does the baby respond to the human voice? Does the baby startle to a loud noise?

Development ▶ Is there a 'social smile'?

Heart and lungs ▶ Is there a heart murmur? Are there signs of heart failure or of respiratory distress?

Abdomen/groins/umbilicus ▶ Is there an abdominal mass or tenderness? Is there a hernia? Is the cord stump healthy?

Hips ▶ Is there evidence of congenital hip dislocation (using Barlow and Ortolani tests; see below)?

Femoral pulses ▶ Are both pulses palpable and of good volume, and in synchrony?

Genitalia ▶ Do the genitalia look normal? Are the labia separate or is there evidence of hypospadias or epispadias. Are both testes palpable in the scrotum?

Spine ▶ Is there a bony defect in the spine? Is there a deep skin pit at the bottom of the spine?

continued

Primitive reflexes ▶ A number of these are normally still present at 6 weeks and can be demonstrated:

▷ *sucking reflex* ▶ the baby sucks vigorously at an object, e.g. a finger, placed in its mouth

▷ *rooting reflex* ▶ the baby's mouth 'roots' or turns towards a stroking motion on its cheek or upper lip, opening its mouth

▷ *Moro reflex* ▶ a defensive reflex of opening the hands and extending and adducting the arms when the baby's head is allowed to 'drop' backwards suddenly or in response to a loud noise. This is also called the startle reflex or parachute reflex (this usually disappears by the age of about 4 months, and is always abnormal if present after the age of 6 months)

▷ *stepping reflex* ▶ the baby lifts its leg in 'a step' when its foot touches a horizontal surface

▷ *grasp reflex* ▶ the baby's hand grips, e.g. a finger or other object placed in its palm, in a primitive grasp (this usually disappears after the age of about 4 months).

The 6-week check

The 6-week check is very similar to the newborn examination, and is accompanied by some screening questions and assessment of growth charts.

Some examples of useful screening questions are given in Box 2.2.

Box 2.2 ○ *Postnatal screening questions*

1 ▷ Do you feel well yourself?
2 ▷ Are there any problems feeding your baby?
3 ▷ Are you pleased with your baby's weight gain?
4 ▷ Does your baby look towards the light?
5 ▷ Does your baby watch you and follow you with his or her eyes?
6 ▷ Does your baby smile at you?
7 ▷ Do you think your baby can hear you?
8 ▷ Is your baby startled by loud noises?
9 ▷ Is your baby easy to look after?
10 ▷ Do you have any worries about your baby?

The first question screens for postnatal depression, as do questions 9 and 10. If there is any suggestion that the baby's mother may have postnatal depression, the next step is the administration of the Edinburgh Postnatal

Depression Screening Questionnaire, which is a validated tool for diagnosing postnatal depression. Questions 2 and 3 are aimed at detecting feeding problems and failure to thrive. Questions 4, 5 and 6 are aimed at detecting problems with vision, and question 6 may also give an indication of developmental problems. Questions 7 and 8 are aimed at detecting problems with hearing, and question 8 may also indicate neurological problems (as 'startling' depends on the hearing of the noise and the intact startle reflex). Question 10 is an open question and allows various concerns to be raised by the mother and addressed. First-time mothers especially may not want to make a specific doctor's appointment but may welcome the opportunity to address various niggling worries.

The 6-week check is a good opportunity to discuss parents' feeling and concerns about immunisations, and to answer any questions they may have. Patient information leaflets have often been given already by the health visitor, who usually visits when the baby is about 11 days old, so the parents should have had time to reflect and to think of questions.

Neonatal screening

Neonatal screening includes blood tests done on a 'heel-prick' blood test, known as the Guthrie test, usually taken by the midwife at 7 days of age. In some areas, neonatal auditory screening is available, although this is often delivered only to babies identified as 'at risk' of hearing problems, such as those with a family history. In many areas, screening by ultrasound assessment of the hips is also offered to babies identified as at 'high risk' of congenital hip dislocation – those born breech or with a family history. However, the costs of administering these tests are significant, and are one reason why these tests are not routinely offered to all infants.

Neonatal screening by blood tests

The blood tests used nationally on the 7-days heel-prick blood sample are shown in Table 2.1:

Table 2.1 ○ **Neonatal screening**

Test	Population
Congenital hypothyroidism	All newborn babies
Cystic fibrosis	All newborn babies

continued

Test	Population
Medium-chain acyl-CoA dehydrogenase deficiency (MCADD)	All newborn babies in England since May 2009
Phenylketonuria (PKU)	All newborn babies
Sickle cell disease and thalassaemia	All newborn babies in high prevalence areas (prevalence of sickle cell > 1.5/10,000 pregnancies)

Neonatal screening of hearing

It is estimated that between one and two children per 1000 live births have a moderate or greater bilateral permanent hearing loss.[3] Pilot schemes have used the automated hearing screen, delivered ideally within the first 7 days after birth. It is likely that this will eventually replace the traditional 'distraction' test, which is performed at 7 to 9 months of age. This is a fairly crude test, usually performed by health visitors, using a Manchester rattle. The baby is 'distracted' from watching a toy and observations made as to whether the baby turns its head towards a rattle shaken to one side out of the line of vision. It is undecided yet whether automated hearing screening will be universal or administered only to a selected 'high risk' population of newborns.

Risk factors for hearing problems include:[4]

▷ a family history of hearing problems
▷ congenital infections, including meningitis
▷ craniofacial abnormalities
▷ low Apgar score
▷ low birthweight
▷ ototoxic drugs
▷ admission to neonatal ITU for > 48 hours.

A study of newborn screening for hearing loss in Germany, published in 2006, compared universal newborn hearing screening (every hospital-born baby screened during the first few days of life), risk factor screening (screening of all children with one or more risk factors for hearing loss) and no systematic screening.[4] By the age of 6 months, universal screening had detected 72.2 per cent, risk factor screening had detected 44.1 per cent and no active screening had detected 17 per cent (percentages of children diagnosed ultimately by age 72 months with definite hearing impairment). Children with congenital hearing impairment benefit from early detection and treatment, as the development of hearing in the brain requires acoustic stimulation in the first 18 months after birth.[5]

One of the difficulties of screening for hearing problems in children is that cohort studies show that the number of confirmed cases of hearing impairment increases with each passing year. This increase continues until the age of 9 years and probably beyond.[6-8] This rise in cumulative prevalence with age is partly due to delayed diagnosis of stable congenital impairments and partly due to delayed onset including acquired impairment (e.g. post-meningitis) and progressive disorders (e.g. post-cytomegalovirus or certain genetic disorders). One study found that the prevalence of confirmed permanent childhood hearing impairment in the UK is possibly two per 1000, although the previous yields from the UK screening programme were only one per 1000.[8,9]

Neonatal screening of hips

Universal clinical screening of the hips for developmental dysplasia of the hip (DDH) was first introduced in the UK in the mid-1960s, although it has never been assessed formally as a screening tool in a randomised controlled trial. The decision to screen was driven historically by the perceived poor outcome for children associated with delay in diagnosis and surgical treatment. There has been considerable debate about this screening, especially as the consequence of false positives being treated unnecessarily is the risk of avascular necrosis of the femoral head.[10] Most studies on DDH screening focus on cost-effectiveness. A recent study[11] attempted to analyse and compare the cost-effectiveness of four strategies:

▷ clinical screening alone (Ortolani and Barlow tests; Figure 2.1)
▷ clinical screening and additional static and dynamic ultrasound examination of the hips of all infants ('universal ultrasound')
▷ clinical screening and additional ultrasound for infants with defined risk factors ('selective ultrasound')
▷ no screening (i.e. clinical diagnosis only).

Ultrasound screening strategies were found to be more effective than clinical screening, but also more costly. The 2003 study estimated that total costs for screening and management for 100,000 live births would be:

▷ £4 million for the universal ultrasound screening group
▷ £3 million for the selective ultrasound screening group
▷ £1 million for clinical screening alone
▷ £0.4 million for the 'no screening' group (this reflects the costs of assessment and management of babies who presented clinically with concerns about the hips, but who were not screened in any way).

The relative efficiency of selective and universal ultrasound was poorly differentiated and really depended on how infants were selected for ultrasound, as well as the expertise of clinical screening examiners.[11]

Some areas are now incorporating ultrasound examinations into their screening strategies in some form, particularly for selected 'high risk' infants. Infants identified in this group include those with a positive Ortolani or Barlow test and/or recognised risk factors for DDH, which include:

▷ breech presentation at delivery
▷ positive family history of DDH.

Clinical tests for developmental dysplasia of the hip

In the Ortolani test, the hips are held symmetrically as shown in Figure 2.1. They are then internally rotated and then externally rotated. Suspicion of DDH is triggered by a 'click' (often more palpable than audible) as the femoral head dislocates backwards out of the acetabulum, and then forwards back into it. The Barlow test is a similar manoeuvre but the hips are not moved simultaneously. Instead, one hand fixes one hip, and the other hand rotates the other hip internally and then externally, and a similar 'click' is felt in possible cases of DDH.

Figure 2.1 ○ *Diagrams of the Ortolani (A) and Barlow (B) tests for DDH*

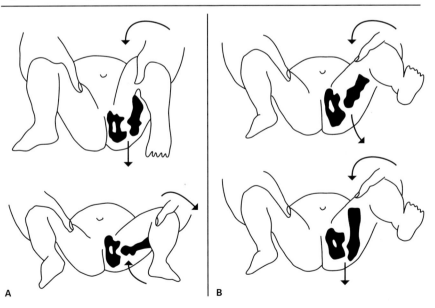

A   B

Other childhood screening

Many regions are phasing in a pre-school vision check by an orthoptist, to replace the check that used to take place in school. In school, children also have a 'sweep' test for hearing (which involves testing hearing at different pitches) and a growth assessment (height and weight).

The previous child health surveillance programme included developmental assessments undertaken by health visitors, in all children at 8 months, 2 years and 3 to 4 years. However, these have now been replaced by a focus on 'at risk' children and families, who are in most need of the health visitor's attention. A recent paper questioned whether the previous child health surveillance programme had contributed to early detection of children with developmental disorders, such as autistic spectrum disorder or speech and language disorder.[12] The paper found that in over 60 per cent of the cases of pervasive developmental disorder detected in 8 to 9-year-olds in the study, there had been documented concerns at the 2-year check, particularly in the area of speech and language development; 94 per cent of the cases had had concerns documented at the three and a half year check, again mainly in the speech and language development area but also increasingly in the behaviour abnormalities area.[12] The researchers concluded that routine surveillance had been a valuable contributing factor for the early detection of pervasive developmental disorders, and suggested that if routine surveillance ceased an alternative method of early detection should be put in place.

Breastfeeding

Midwives, health visitors and other healthcare professionals promote breastfeeding as the optimum way of nourishing a baby. Human breast milk has the ideal combination of proteins, carbohydrates and fats for the growing baby, and is associated with several documented health benefits, such as the following.

Advantages to the baby

The advantages are:

▷ reduced risk of infections in early life (especially gastroenteritis, chest infections and ear infections). Antibodies and proteins are passed down in the breast milk from mother to baby
▷ reduced risk of cot death (possibly secondary to reduced risk of infections)

▷ enhancement of the 'bonding process' between mother and baby, which may affect babies in a positive way emotionally, and even (according to one study) with respect to intelligence[13]

▷ many advantages to the baby's long-term health, e.g. reduction in obesity, less likelihood of hypertension, less likelihood of hypercholesterolaemia, less likelihood of diabetes, leukaemia, asthma and eczema.

In addition there are also advantages to the mother:

▷ convenience
▷ financial
▷ other health benefits, which include reduction in risk of breast cancer, ovarian cancer, Type 2 diabetes and postnatal depression.

It seems these advantages to mother and baby are fully realised after 6 months of exclusive breastfeeding, but there is still some benefit even in babies breastfed for a shorter time or in babies who are partially breastfed.

Despite the encouragement of healthcare professionals and efforts of charities such as the National Childbirth Trust and La Leche League there is a group of women who struggle to breastfeed successfully. These women appear to suffer from excessive suction trauma to the delicate skin of the nipples, making breast-feeding very painful. If genuinely motivated to breastfeed, these difficulties can cause the women to be demoralised, and this often becomes tangled up with feelings of guilt and postnatal depression. These women require sympathetic support with their breastfeeding and sometimes need to introduce formula milk as a supplement and continue to do 'mixed feeding' for as long as they are able.

There are also a few women whose babies fail to thrive in spite of breast-feeding on demand. Although advice such as increasing the mother's fluid intake and improving her diet etc. may help to increase milk production, these women sometimes also need to add formula feeds to ensure that the babies do not miss out on calories and nutrition vital for growth and development.

Meanwhile, a significant number of women opt to bottle-feed from choice from birth onwards or sometimes after some initial problems with breast-feeding. Reasons sometimes cited include:

▷ wanting to include the baby's father in the feeding process
▷ embarrassment when feeding out of the home
▷ not wanting the commitment and 'tie' of breastfeeding
▷ the need to return to work after a short maternity leave
▷ complications such as mastitis that make breastfeeding very painful.

The Office for National Statistics performs its Infant Feeding Survey every 5 years. The 2005 figures were published in March 2008 and showed some significant findings:[14]

▷ the proportion of babies breastfed at birth in the UK rose by 7 per cent

▷ Scotland, which showed the greatest increases in the prevalence of breastfeeding at ages up to 9 months in 2000, appears to have stabilised in 2005, with a small increase in the rate at 4 months and no increase at 6 and 9 months. By contrast, the other UK countries show an increase at all these ages

▷ overall, only 35 per cent of UK babies are being exclusively breastfed at 1 week, 21 per cent at 6 weeks, 7 per cent at 4 months and 3 per cent at 5 months.

Information Services Division (ISD) Scotland figures show that a number of personal, social and cultural issues is strongly associated with the likelihood of breastfeeding, including maternal age, deprivation and smoking status.[15] Data are collected from 11 NHS Board areas, accounting for 89 per cent of Scotland's pre-school population. Key points for the data include:

▷ in 2007, almost 45 per cent of mothers were breastfeeding at around 10 days (this included 37.5 per cent of mothers who were exclusively breastfeeding and 7 per cent who were doing 'mixed feeding'). This was very similar to the 2006 figures

▷ at the 6- to 8-week review, the overall breastfeeding rate was 36 per cent in 2007, which included 26.4 per cent exclusively breastfeeding and 9.6 per cent mixed feeding. These figures were also very similar to the 2006 figures

▷ the overall breastfeeding and exclusive breastfeeding rates have remained relatively stable since 2001

▷ breastfeeding rates vary across NHS Board areas, e.g. at the 6- to 8-week review, exclusive breastfeeding rates in 2007 ranged from 18.8 per cent in Ayrshire and Arran to 35 per cent in Lothian.

The ISD Scotland breastfeeding data also demonstrate that personal, social and cultural issues are strongly associated with the likelihood of breastfeeding.[15] The most important of these factors are:

▷ **maternal age** ▶ older mothers are more likely to breastfeed than younger mothers. In 2007, only 5.9 per cent of mothers under age 20 were exclusively breastfeeding at 6 to 8 weeks, compared with 37.7 per cent of mothers aged 40 and over

▷ **social deprivation** ▶ mothers in the least deprived areas are three times more likely to exclusively breastfeed at 6 to 8 weeks than mothers in the most deprived areas (42.3 per cent compared with 13.9 per cent respectively)

▷ **smoking** ▶ non-smoking mothers are nearly three times as likely to exclusively breastfeed their babies by around 10 days of age, as mothers who smoke. In 2007, 43.3 per cent of non-smoking mothers exclusively breastfed their babies, compared with 15.4 per cent of mothers who smoked.

There are also interesting relationships between these factors, e.g. the positive effect of maternal age on breastfeeding is less pronounced in more deprived areas. The combination of these two factors results in an even greater divide in breastfeeding statistics, with only 5 per cent of younger mothers (age 20 and below) in the most deprived areas exclusively breast-feeding at 6 to 8 weeks, compared with 50.9 per cent of mothers aged 40 and over in the least deprived areas, for children born between 2001 and 2007.

Immunisations

The UK immunisation schedule

The current UK immunisation schedule is shown in Table 2.2 (p. 26). It has been subject to a number of changes over recent years, which include:

▷ the introduction of Hib (*Haemophilus influenzae* type B) immunisation, which protects young children against epiglottitis and meningitis
▷ meningitis C immunisation, introduced to protect babies from *Neisseria meningitidis* C
▷ the introduction in 2006 of pneumococcal vaccine, to protect against strains of streptococcus, which can cause meningitis or pneumonia in babies
▷ the introduction in 2008 of human papillomavirus (HPV) immunisation at the age of 12–13 years in girls, to protect against the two strains of HPV most likely to cause cervical cancer (this programme is discussed further in Chapter 13).

There has also been considerable debate about the measles, mumps and rubella (MMR) immunisation, which is offered at the age of 13 months, with a booster at the age of 3 years. The debate was sparked off in 1998 by a study from the Royal Free Hospital, in which paediatric gastroenterologist Andrew Wakefield suggested that administering separate monovalent measles, mumps and rubella vaccines might be less likely to cause autism or inflammatory bowel disease than administration of the combined MMR vaccine. Given extensive media coverage this issue led to a situation of near panic among parents who requested that the NHS should give parents the choice of single or combined administration of the MMR vaccines. However, the government, advised by the Chief Medical Officer, refused to offer the 'single vaccines' on the NHS, not least because this would entail a course of six injections rather than the two injections of MMR, and compliance with the complete course was very likely to be poor compared with compliance with the combined MMR immunisation. Public concern about the combined MMR vaccination led to a significant drop in MMR immunisation rates over a period of several years, and some outbreaks of measles and mumps in areas of low vaccine uptake. It was often the parents from higher social classes who refused the combined MMR vaccine, opting instead to either pay privately for the single vaccines or to watch and wait for further advice to be published.

Further research has demonstrated not only the efficacy of the MMR but also its safety. Large studies in various countries, including the UK and Japan, have failed to show any significant risk of autism or inflammatory bowel disease in association with the MMR vaccine.

The current UK immunisation schedule, 2008–9, is shown in Table 2.2:

Table 2.2 ○ **UK immunisation schedule**[16]

3 days	1. BCG (if tuberculosis (TB) in family in last 6 months, see also Box 2.3) 2. Hepatitis B vaccine if mother is HBsAg +ve	
2 months	1. Diphtheria, tetanus, pertussis, polio and Haemophilus influenzae type b (DTaP/IPV/Hib) 2. Pneumococcal (PCV)	1. One injection (pediacel) 2. One injection (prevenar)
3 months	1. Diphtheria, tetanus, pertussis, polio and Haemophilus influenzae type b (DTaP/IPV/Hib) 2. Meningitis C (MenC)	1. One injection (pediacel) 2. One injection (neisvac C or meningitec)
4 months	1. Diphtheria, tetanus, pertussis, polio and Haemophilus influenzae type b (DTaP/IPV/Hib) 2. Pneumococcal (PCV) 3. Meningitis C (MenC)	1. One injection (pediacel) 2. One injection (prevenar) 3. One injection (neisvac C or meningitec)

continued

Around 12 months	*Haemophilus influenzae* type b, meningitis C (Hib/MenC)	One injection (menitorix)
Around 13 months	1. Measles, mumps and rubella (MMR) 2. Pneumococcal (PCV)	1. One injection (priorix or MMR II) 2. One injection (prevenar)
3 years and 4 months or soon after	1. Diphtheria, tetanus, pertussis and polio (DTaP/IPV) 2. Measles, mumps and rubella (MMR)	1. One injection (repevax or infanrix-IPV) 2. One injection (priorix or MMR II)
13–18 years	Tetanus, diphtheria and polio (Td/IPV)	One injection (revaxis)

In addition, the national policy is that influenza vaccine and one-off pneumococcal vaccination should be offered to all those aged 6 months or over in a clinical risk group.

There have been some recent changes to the national immunisation screening programme involving adolescents. The Heaf test and BCG vaccination are no longer routinely carried out in all adolescents, but only in those who are identified as at high risk (see Box 2.3). BCG vaccination is now included in the childhood immunisation programme for high-risk babies so it is anticipated that administration of BCG in adolescents will gradually fall.

Box 2.3 ○ *UK immunisation against TB with the BCG vaccine*

1 ▷ Babies living in areas of the UK where there is a high rate of TB. That is, areas where the incidence of TB is 40 cases per 100,000 people per year, or greater.

2 ▷ Babies whose parents or grandparents have lived in a country with a high rate of TB. That is, countries where the incidence of TB is 40 cases per 100,000 people per year, or greater.

Adolescents in the following groups who have not previously been immunised:

3 ▷ Immigrants to the UK from countries where TB is common.

4 ▷ Close contacts of people with active TB.

5 ▷ People who intend to live for 1 month or more in countries with a high TB rate.

Until 2005, all schoolchildren in the UK were routinely given the BCG vaccine at about the age of 13. The policy changed in autumn 2005 due to the changing patterns of TB in the UK. Rates of the disease are now very low in many parts of the country and children living in these areas have a very small risk of infection. However, in other areas, rates of TB are increasing. This is why the BCG vaccine is now mainly targeted at babies living in areas where there is an increasing rate of TB cases. Those children who would previously have been offered BCG through the schools' programme will now be screened for risk factors, tested and immunised as appropriate.

There are several considerations to be taken into account with immunisations:

1 ▷ An acute febrile illness is a contraindication to any vaccine
2 ▷ Give live vaccines either together, or separated by ≥ 3 weeks
3 ▷ Proceed with caution with live vaccines in patients who are immune deficient (transplants, cancer chemotherapy, HIV infection) – seek expert advice
4 ▷ Target at-risk group for influenza and/or pneumococcal vaccination.

Summary of key points

▷ The current UK child health promotion programme includes screening examinations within the first 24 hours and at 6 weeks of age.
▷ Screening tests using heel-prick blood tests are national, but subject to local variations in specific policies.
▷ Screening tests for senses such as vision and hearing are subject to local policies and are currently still being phased in.
▷ There are still no routine screening tests for many speech, language, developmental and congenital disorders.
▷ Children at high risk of certain conditions may need additional screening tests
▷ If a parent suspects a problem with his or her child, HE OR SHE IS OFTEN RIGHT! The views and concerns of parents and other carers should always be taken seriously.

How does the GP curriculum help us think about the care of this group of patients?

Primary care management

All children are currently invited for neonatal screening blood tests and examinations (at birth and at 6 weeks), and for immunisations according to the national immunisation programme. The GP and the primary care team often know other family members and may even have known the mother as a child. This background helps the GP understand the social context into which a baby is born.

Person-centred care

Further screening tests often depend on an assessment of a child's individual risk factors for specific conditions.

Specific problem-solving skills

The role of primary care is to identify children at risk of problems or with evidence to suggest that a problem may be present. Referral to secondary care may be required for specific diagnoses.

A comprehensive approach

The GP is in an ideal position to co-ordinate health promotion services and ensure that interventions are undertaken when appropriate. The hand-held child record (red book) is a useful tool in this.

Community orientation

The GP is part of a mutually supportive multidisciplinary team in primary care, and works alongside midwives, health visitors, social workers and community paediatricians.

A holistic approach

This is the desired outcome, and can be achieved with good teamwork focusing on the individual needs of each child and family.

Box 2.4 ○ **Child health promotion check**

Consider the case of a 6-week-old breastfed baby who comes for its routine child health promotion check. Mum says that the baby screams to feed and then struggles and fights. She has noticed a tongue-tie and wonders if it is relevant. What would you do?

The growth chart is reproduced in Figure 2.2 showing that the baby has clearly fallen from the 50th centile line to the 2nd centile.

The baby is not vomiting, has no diarrhoea, is desperately hungry and yet struggles to feed.

continued

This is a real case, and the baby was referred urgently to a paediatric surgeon, and the tongue tie was snipped under general anaesthesia. The baby started to feed hungrily as soon as the site started to heal and within a week the slope of the growth chart had turned itself around and the baby started to thrive.

Some cases of tongue tie will have no impact on a baby's ability to feed. Some of these may affect speech and language development, whilst others will have no deleterious impact at all. The problem should be treated according to the impact it is having on the baby.

In this case, we see the need for regular weight monitoring. This is useful for any breastfed baby (where there is no way to be sure how much milk is being ingested) and where there is a query about weight gain. It is especially true in firstborn babies, where mothers may be less confident and will have no experience of previous breastfeeding.

Figure 2.2 ○ *Growth chart for a baby boy aged 6 weeks*

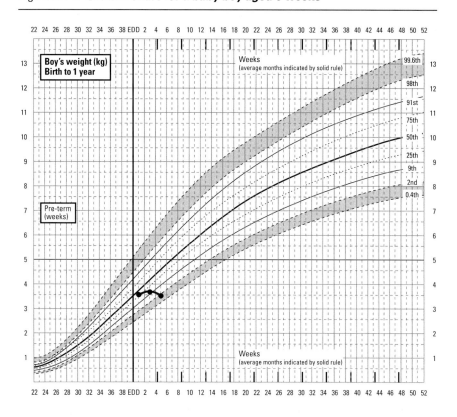

Source: © Child Growth Foundation.

References

1 • Secretaries of State for Health, Wales, Northern Ireland and Scotland. *Working for Patients* London: DoH, 1990.

2 • Department of Health. *National Service Framework for Children, Young People and Maternity Services* London: DoH, 2004.

3 • Parving A, Hauch A M. Permanent childhood hearing impairment: some cross-sectional characteristics from a surveillance programme *International Pediatrics* 2001; **16(1)**: 1–5.

4 • Grill E, Hessel F, Siebert U, *et al.* Comparing the clinical effectiveness of different new-born hearing screening strategies: a decision analysis *BMC Public Health* 2005; **5**: 12–22.

5 • Yoshinaga-Itano C, Sedey A L, Coulter D K, *et al.* Language of early- and later-identified children with hearing loss *Pediatrics* 1998; **102(5)**: 1161–71.

6 • Upfold I, Isepy J. Childhood deafness in Australia: incidence and maternal rubella 1949–1980 *Medical Journal of Australia* 1982; **2(7)**: 323–6.

7 • Parving A, Christensen B. Epidemiology of permanent hearing impairment on children in relation to costs of a hearing health surveillance programme *International Journal of Pediatric Otorhinolaryngology* 1996; **3**: 9-23.

8 • Fortnum H M, Summerfield A Q, Marshall D H, *et al.* Prevalence of permanent hearing impairment in the United Kingdom and implications for universal neonatal hearing screening: questionnaire-based ascertainment study *British Medical Journal* 2001; **323(7312)**: 536–40.

9 • Wessex Universal Hearing Screening Trial Group. Controlled trial of universal neonatal screening for early identification of permanent childhood hearing impairment *Lancet* 1998; **352**: 1957–64.

10 • Dezateux C, Brown J, Arthur R, *et al.* Performance, treatment pathways and effects of alternative policy options for screening for developmental dysplasia of the hip in the United Kingdom *Archives of Diseases in Childhood* 2003; **88**: 753–9.

11 • Brown J, Dezateux C, Karnon J, *et al.* Efficiency of alternative policy options for screening for developmental dysplasia of the hip in the United Kingdom *Archives of Diseases in Childhood* 2003; **88**: 760–6.

12 • Tebruegge M, Nandini V, Ritchie J. Does routine child health surveillance contribute to the early detection of children with pervasive developmental disorders? An epidemiological study in Kent, UK *BMC Pediatrics* 2004; **4(4)**: 1–7.

13 • Der G, Batty G D, Deary I J. Effect of breastfeeding on intelligence in children: prospective study, sibling pairs analysis, and meta-analysis *British Medical Journal* 2006; **333**: 945–8.

14 • www.babyfriendly.org.uk [accessed August 2009].

15 • www.isdscotland.org/isd/5637.html [accessed August 2009].

16 • Department of Health. *Important Changes to the Childhood Immunisation Programme* London: DoH, 2006.

Child health promotion

Vince Ion

3

Introduction

In this chapter, we look at the opportunities that working with a wider range of healthcare professionals can bring to promote child health, and also at the wider opportunities for family health.

The key members of the primary care team working with the general practitioner (GP) to promote child health are midwives, health visitors, practice and school nurses. Working as a team they can make a significant impact on educating families to promote a healthy lifestyle. This in turn can reduce the risks to children and families of the major chronic diseases such as diabetes and coronary heart disease. Opportunities for health education on issues such as immunisation, accident prevention, nutrition, smoking, and alcohol and substance misuse can be best approached working in teams.

Primary care teams are best placed to understand their locality challenges. Some of the key elements in promoting child health will be the need to adapt advice and approach where there is a range of ethnic communities. For example, the risk of diabetes, obesity and hypertension is greater in people of South Asian, Caribbean and West African origin than in the white population of the UK. The need and opportunity to target such communities is therefore a potential priority for health promotion.

Scenario

To set the scene, think about the following scenario. You are seeing a young family that includes a child who is starting school in the next 6 months and a newborn baby. They have recently moved into the area and you have very little history about the family at this appointment.

▷ *Consider what your priorities are for this family. Who else in the primary care team would you include in the management of these priorities?*

The RCGP curriculum outcomes

The competent practitioner: [1]

▷ promotes health and wellbeing by applying health promotion and disease prevention strategies appropriately, and detects problems that may already be present but have not yet been detected. He or she will be aware of a GP's role in:
  ▶ promoting and organising immunisation
  ▶ the prevention of accidents
▷ works effectively with colleagues across professional boundaries
▷ recognises inequalities and ethnic diversity, and addresses them proactively
▷ manages simultaneously both acute and chronic problems in the child, young person and family by:
  ▶ assessing children and young people's developmental needs in the context of their family and environmental factors, including school and community, and parenting capacity
  ▶ understanding the key vulnerability factors for children and young people in special circumstances and responding to their needs, including through referral and joint working
▷ refers to the health visitor and other professionals for a comprehensive family needs assessment to understand and address the impact of the parents' needs on the children's health and development.

The role and responsibilities of the health visitor

The role of the health visiting team is to deliver measurable health outcomes for individuals and communities.[2] Health visitors will also play a significant role in meeting the Department of Health standards in the National Service Framework (NSF).[3]

The health visitor is a qualified registered nurse, midwife, sick children's nurse or psychiatric nurse with specialist qualifications in community health, which includes child health, health promotion and education. A health visitor's role is a varied one and is an integral part of the primary care team. The main focus of his or her work is prevention – helping people and families to stay healthy and avoid illness.

The role involves promoting health in the whole community and health visitors are particularly involved with families who have children under 5 and with the elderly population. Because most are attached to GP practices they can work with all registered patients. They look at the broader picture to identify the health needs within their community and this means they have a key role, if consulted, in affecting local policy.

Every family with children under 5 has a named health visitor. The role here is to offer support and encouragement to families through the early years from pregnancy and birth to primary school and beyond.

Help and advice

Health visitors can provide help and advice to parents on the following topics:

▷ the growth and development of the child
▷ common infections in childhood
▷ common skin problems
▷ behaviour difficulties – sleeping, eating, potty training, temper tantrums and teething
▷ breastfeeding, weaning, healthy eating, hygiene, safety and exercise
▷ postnatal depression advice, advice for bereavement and violence in the family.

They are also involved in:

▷ working in partnership with families to tailor health plans to their needs
▷ co-ordinating child immunisation programmes
▷ organising and running baby clinics
▷ health promotion groups, breastfeeding support groups, parent support groups, parenting courses
▷ nurse prescribing.

Working with fathers is a difficult area for all health professionals.[4] Even a father in a family that lives together can be the 'silent partner', as often fathers will be at work during the Monday to Friday routine of general practice.

Where fathers are either working away of are living separately from their children then this 'silent partner' element can be further exaggerated. Using this as an example of potential social isolation, the work of the health visitor can be significant in supporting fathers and families, ensuring that they have the opportunity to engage fully in their role as a parent. This may however mean thinking of different ways of how, when and where to offer services to families, including engaging in conjunction with midwives and the prenatal care of families, and asking families a range of questions on this issue.

When to work with the primary care team

It is necessary to ensure that all fathers have the opportunity to contribute to how they see their role in the prenatal and postnatal period. Consider what action is needed and how to identify the priorities for fathers and their families. Who else in the primary care team and beyond should be consulted? Who should lead on this, and why?

Immunisation

Consider the following: the new practice nurse phones you to say that she has a mother in her surgery. This patient has brought a raft of information about the immunisation of her baby, which she has looked up on the web. She has many questions about the balance of risk and benefit.

The nurse is unsure how to respond to the mother. How would you proceed? What advice would you offer?

Immunisation and vaccination programmes are an excellent example of a primary preventive approach to reduce or eliminate the infectious diseases of childhood such as whooping cough, measles, rubella, poliomyelitis and mumps, which can have serious consequences.[5]

The current UK immunisation schedule is outlined in Chapter 2.

Specific preventive initiatives will often be used in combination with other health promotion activities. In the example of immunisation, health education is essential to raise parents' awareness of the benefits of immunisation and encourage them to use this programme. It is useful to have a multi-professional approach to such health education within the primary care team.

The immunisation programme for a number of years has come under some scrutiny by parents following a range of media publicity about the measles, mumps and rubella (MMR) programme in particular. This has meant a reduction of uptake of this and some other elements of the programme. To manage this effectively an agreed approach across all professionals is needed so that parents receive consistent advice that is in line with the agreed national policy.

Holistic assessment and early interventions for young people and their families

To offer a holistic assessment of any person is always a goal for those working within the primary care team. The aim is to support transition periods, to maximise children's achievements and opportunities, and understand their rights and responsibilities.[1] This goal can be difficult to achieve for a range of reasons. This includes engagement of the young person, environmental barriers such as surgery and clinic times clashing with school, the time involved and the need for a multi-professional/agency approach.

The common assessment framework (CAF) is a key part of delivering frontline services that are integrated and focused around the needs of children and young people. The CAF is a standardised approach to conducting an assessment of a child's additional needs and deciding how those needs should be met. It can be used by practitioners across children's services in England and Wales.[6]

The CAF will promote more effective, earlier identification of additional needs, particularly in universal services. It is intended to provide a simple process for a holistic assessment of a child's needs and strengths, taking account the role of parents, carers and environmental factors on its development. Practitioners will then be better placed to agree, with the child and family, about what support is appropriate. The CAF will also help to improve integrated working by promoting co-ordinated service provision.[7]

GPs' professional backgrounds may define their patterns of thought and action; medical personnel have a scientific training that may be substantially different from that of nurses, health visitors, teachers and social workers. Unless GPs spend time with any of these groups of professionals they have little shared understanding of the paradigms in which everyone functions.

Multi-professional working can be extremely helpful in bringing about a shared understanding between professionals dealing with children.[7] The emergence of children's centres, Sure Start and other support provided in the wider context of public health outside of a GP practice is helpful in bringing non-health agencies and health professionals together. This may be a setting that can be seen by the child and its family as less intimidating. However, it is also possible for such work to move forward positively in any setting.

General practice in the UK is characterised by the relationship, over time, between doctor, patient and family.[8] GPs can be protective of this relationship; however, the requirements of a holistic assessment are best delivered by all those involved in the primary care team working together.

Early health promotion interventions to address the needs of children and families

The health promotion services that will be offered to all pregnant women and children are identified in the first standard in the *National Service Framework for Children, Young People and Maternity Services:*[3]

The health and well-being of all children and young people is promoted and delivered through a co-ordinated programme of action, including prevention and early intervention wherever possible, to ensure long term gain, led by the NHS in partnership with local authorities.

It is designed to be delivered across the primary care team. Details can be found online at www.dh.gov.uk/en/Publicationsandstatistics/Publications/PublicationsPolicyAndGuidance/Browsable/DH_4865614.

Markers of good practice for this standard are given in Box 3.1.

Box 3.1 ○ *Markers of good practice under standard 1 of the* National Service Framework for Children, Young People and Maternity Services

1 ▷ The Child Health Promotion Programme is offered to all children and young people and their families in a range of settings.

2 ▷ By the child's first birthday, a systematic assessment of its physical, emotional and social development and family needs is carried out. Information resulting from assessments and interventions is recorded in the 'red book'.

3 ▷ Screening and immunisation programmes within the Child Health Promotion Programme are delivered to all children through partnership working.

4 ▷ Where there are concerns about a child or young person's health and development, parents receive timely and effective assessment and response.

5 ▷ Therapy services are available for all children and young people who require them, and systems are in place to minimise waiting times for access to these services.

6 ▷ Health promotion, in terms of awareness-raising, information-giving and support services, including the Child Health Promotion Programme, is reflected in improved outcomes for children and young people.

7 ▷ All schools work towards becoming part of the Healthy Schools Programme, and are responsive to their school population's needs.

8 ▷ Primary care trusts and local authorities tailor health promotion services to the needs of disadvantaged groups, including children in special circumstances, identified through a local population needs assessment.

Confidentiality within teams

The larger the healthcare team becomes, the harder it can be to determine where its boundaries are and what information can legitimately be shared. At times, most health professionals have struggled to know how much of what is learned in a conversation can be shared with colleagues, particularly in other agencies. For GP trainees worried about involving health visitors and others, in child protection issues for example, the General Medical Council (GMC) has issued guidance on the issue, reinforcing the absolute need to share information. In England and Wales, the Children Acts of 1989 and 2004 give GPs a statutory duty to share information if there are concerns about a child's safety or welfare (section 47 and section 27, duty to co-operate, Children Act 1989).[9] The GMC states:[10]

Your first concern must be the safety of children and young people. You must inform an appropriate person or authority promptly of any reasonable concern that children or young people are at risk of abuse or neglect, when that is in a child's best interests or necessary to protect other children or young people. You must be able to justify a decision not to share such a concern.

The doctor must:

▷ remember and understand the procedures and legislation relating to confidentiality issues that apply to his or her job role
▷ understand the limits of confidentiality that apply to his or her job role. It is sometimes necessary to go against children's or young people's expressed wishes in their best interests. Where this is the case, the GP must ensure that they understand what is happening and why.

However, this still leaves questions about the duty of confidentiality due to other family members. The GP is responsible for ensuring that any disclosure of information is justified by the risk to a child or young person, that it is proportionate to the situation, and that the reasons for disclosure or non-disclosure are well-recorded. Guidance on this may be sought from the UK Defence Organisations.[11]

An example of team working

Consider the following scenario: the receptionist tells you that a couple has made an appointment to see you next week to discuss Sudden Infant Death (SID). They have previously had a cot death in the family and are worried about the possibility of a familial link to SIDs.

How would you offer advice and support on this issue? Who else within the primary care team may also be able to offer help? The following information might be useful.

Sudden Infant Death

Cot death is a term commonly used to describe a sudden and unexpected infant death that is initially unexplained. Cot deaths that remain unexplained after a thorough examination are usually registered as SIDs. All healthcare professionals will find this subject difficult to discuss with a family.

A thorough post-mortem examination will reveal a specific cause of death in less than half of all cot deaths. Causes may include accidents, infection, congenital abnormality or metabolic disorder. For the cases that remain unexplained (SIDs) researchers think there are likely to be undiscovered causes. For many it is likely that a combination of factors affect a baby at a vulnerable stage of development.

Features of cot death[12]

Cot death can occur anywhere and at any time. Although cot deaths do usually occur during a period of sleep in the cot, babies can die during any other period of sleep, e.g. in their parent's arms or in a pram.

When babies are found dead in their parents' bed or with their faces covered it is sometimes thought they have died from suffocation. It is not known how often suffocation is in fact a total explanation for the baby's death. Cot death can affect any baby. However, certain babies are more at risk, namely: premature babies; low birthweight babies; boys; and babies born to young mothers who already have other children.

Cot death is uncommon in babies less than a month old, but rises to a peak during the second month. The risk then diminishes as the baby grows older. Nearly 90 per cent of cot deaths have occurred by 6 months, and very few occur after a year.

Cot death can happen to any family, though it is more frequent in families who live in difficult circumstances or who smoke a lot. It is uncommon in Asian families, for reasons that are not yet understood. It is very rare for cot death to occur twice in the same family, though occasionally an inherited disorder, such as a metabolic defect, may cause more than one infant to die unexpectedly.

How can the risk of cot death be reduced?

The following advice can be offered to families:

▷ cut smoking in pregnancy and do not let anyone smoke in the same room as the baby, including all family members and friends
▷ always place the baby on its back to sleep
▷ do not let the baby get too hot
▷ place the baby with its feet to the foot of the cot, to prevent it wriggling down under the covers
▷ never sleep with the baby on a sofa or armchair
▷ the safest place for the baby to sleep is in a crib or cot in a room with the parent(s) for the first 6 months.

It is especially dangerous for the baby to sleep in the parents' bed if one or more of the parents:

▷ is a smoker, even if he or she never smokes in bed or at home
▷ has been drinking alcohol
▷ takes medication or drugs that cause drowsiness
▷ feels very tired

or if the baby:

▷ was born before 37 weeks
▷ weighed less than 2.5 kg or 5½ lbs at birth
▷ is less than 3 months old.

Do not forget that accidents can happen. A parent might roll over during sleep and suffocate the baby, or the baby could get caught between the wall and the bed, or could roll out of an adult bed and be injured. Settling the baby to sleep (day and night) with a dummy can reduce the risk of cot death, even if the dummy falls out while the baby is asleep. The mother should breastfeed the baby, and establish breastfeeding before starting to use a dummy.

Support for parents who have had a cot death and are having another baby

The Care of the Next Infant (CONI) programme, run by the Foundation for the Study of Infant Deaths in conjunction with the NHS, is available in 91 per cent of the country. This scheme offers advice, support and practical help to cot death parents in the care of their next baby.

The rate of SIDs remained fairly constant, at about 2 per 1000 live births, from 1971 to 1988, and then began to decline. The rate has fallen by around

41

75 per cent since the Reduce the Risk campaign was launched in 1991. However, 300 babies died suddenly and unexpectedly in the UK in 2005 making cot death the largest kind of death in babies over 1 month old.

Cot death in comparison with other childhood problems and in other countries

Cot death remains the most common kind of death in babies aged over 1 month old. Far more babies die as cot deaths each year than from road traffic accidents, leukaemia and meningitis put together.

It is similar to countries such as France, Norway and Sweden. The rate is lower in the Netherlands and Japan, but higher in New Zealand, Australia and the USA. In recent years the rate in many industrialised countries has declined, as in the UK, following the introduction of Reduce the Risk campaigns.

The opportunity to work in collaboration and across health professions is also an opportunity to ensure that consistent and repeated advice is offered to all families on this subject.

Top tips on child health promotion

▷ Work as a team.
▷ Have a lead within the practice for child health promotion.
▷ Identify the key themes the primary care team will focus on and ensure the whole team knows them.
▷ Have clear objectives and priorities with regard to health promotion.
▷ Have training available for all staff.
▷ Ensure that the practice and services are children- and young person-friendly.
▷ Have an easily accessible list of other resources available to families on health promotion.
▷ Have regular meetings to review the latest key issues in relation to health promotion.

Web resources

▷ Doctors.net, electronic Continuing Medical Education (eCME), **www.doctors.net.uk** [accessed August 2009].
▷ NHS immunisation information, **www.immunisation.nhs.uk** [accessed August 2009].

▷ Department for Children, Schools and Families,
www.dcsf.gov.uk/index.htm [accessed August 2009].

▷ Nutrition Subcommittee of the Diabetes Care Advisory Committee. *The Implementation of Nutritional Advice for People with Diabetes*, 2003, **www.diabetes.org.uk/Documents/Professionals/nutrition_guidelines.pdf** [accessed August 2009].

▷ General Medical Council. *0–18 years: guidance for all doctors* London: GMC, 2007, **www.gmc-uk.org/guidance/ethical_guidance/children_guidance/index.asp** [accessed August 2009].

References

1 • Royal College of General Practitioners. *Care of Children and Young People* (curriculum statement 8) London: RCGP, 2007, www.rcgp-curriculum.org.uk/pdf/curr_8_Care_of_Children_and_Young_People.pdf [accessed August 2009].

2 • Department of Health. *Facing the Future: a review of the role of the Health Visitor* London: TSO, 2007, www.dh.gov.uk/en/Publicationsandstatistics/Publications/PublicationsPolicyAndGuidance/DH_075642 [accessed August 2009].

3 • Department for Education and Skills, Department of Health. *National Service Framework for Children, Young People and Maternity Services: core standards* London: DoH, 2004, www.dh.gov.uk/en/Publicationsandstatistics/Publications/PublicationsPolicyAndGuidance/DH_4089099 [accessed August 2009].

4 • Ryan M. *Working with Fathers* Abingdon: Radcliffe Medical Press, 2000.

5 • Donaldson RJ, Donaldson LJ. *Essential Public Health Medicine* Abingdon: Radcliffe Medical Press, 2000.

6 • Department of Health. *Every Child Matters: common assessment framework*, 2006, www.everychildmatters.gov.uk/deliveringservices/caf/ [accessed August 2009].

7 • Carter Y, Bannon M, Limbert C, *et al.* Improving child protection: a systematic review of training and procedural interventions *Archives of Disease in Childhood* 2006; **91(9)**: 740–3.

8 • Royal College of General Practitioners. *The Future Direction of General Practice: a roadmap* London: RCGP, 2007, www.rcgp.org.uk/pdf/Roadmap_embargoed%20 11am%2013%20Sept.pdf [accessed August 2009].

9 • Children Act 1989, Sections 27 and 47.

10 • General Medical Council. *0–18 years: guidance for all doctors* London: GMC, 2007, www.gmc-uk.org/guidance/ethical_guidance/children_guidance/index.asp [accessed August 2009].

11 • Medical and Dental Defence Union of Scotland. *Essential Guide to Confidentiality* Glasgow: MDDUS, 2007.

12 • The Foundation for the Study of Infant Deaths (FSID), www.sids.org.uk [accessed August 2009].

43

Keeping children and young people safe

4

Andrew Mowat

Introduction

In this chapter, we consider the problems that face us in safeguarding children and young people from harm, and promoting their wellbeing. We examine the prevalence and types of abuse, the factors putting children at risk, the importance of recognition and response to abuse, difficulties presented in consultations relating to safeguarding, confidentiality, working with families and other agencies to make a child safe, and we think through what safeguarding means to the primary care team.

Curriculum outcomes

The competent practitioner will:[1]

▷ utilise the primary care consultation to bring about an effective doctor–child–family relationship
▷ work effectively with colleagues across professional boundaries
▷ work with children and young people, respecting their autonomy
▷ work with families, recognising the child-focused nature of safeguarding but also the value of the family unit
▷ deal effectively with abuse of children and young people by
  ▶ recognising signs of abuse
  ▶ responding appropriately to disclosures of abuse
  ▶ recording clinical observations clearly
  ▶ referring to appropriate agencies
▷ provide continuity of care to meet the needs of the child or young person and family.

Additional competences exist for general practitioners working within the GP with a Special Interest (GPwSIs) scheme.[2]

Safeguarding children – objectives

In *Every Child Matters*,[3] the government sets out its ambitions for every child in the UK:

▷ stay safe
▷ be healthy
▷ enjoy and achieve
▷ make a positive contribution
▷ achieve economic wellbeing.

Safeguarding children and young people is a much wider field than child protection alone. It also involves helping children to achieve these ambitions.

Although there have been improvements in the way in which primary care responds to safeguarding, there are still criticisms[4] of lack of staff training, and lack of support from primary care trusts (PCTs).

Types of abuse

In most UK jurisdictions four different categories of abuse[5,6] are recognised:

▷ physical:
  ▶ may involve hitting, shaking, throwing, poisoning, burning or scalding, drowning, suffocating, or otherwise causing physical harm to a child
  ▶ may be caused when a parent or carer feigns symptoms of, or deliberately causes ill health to, a child he or she is looking after (fabricated or induced illness]
  ▶ features might include:
    ☐ unusual bruising (face, mouth, ears, fingertip pattern, extensive, toolmark)
    ☐ burns (perineum, head, genitalia, hands, legs, feet, glove/stocking, cigarette)
    ☐ cigarette burns may have 'comet tail' where the child has withdrawn from pain
    ☐ bites (human are crescent shape)
    ☐ fractures (reluctance to move a limb, limping, swelling)
    ☐ suffocation, submersion or poisoning (may present as fits or 'funny turns')

▷ emotional
  ▶ persistent emotional ill-treatment of child
  ▶ severe/persistent bad effect on child's emotional development
  ▶ may involve
    ☐ making child feel worthless or unloved
    ☐ inadequate or valued only to meet needs of another person
    ☐ causing children to feel frightened
    ☐ exploitation or corruption of children
    ☐ age or developmentally inappropriate expectations imposed on children
  ▶ features vary according to age, and might include:
    ☐ physical (failure to thrive, infection, nappy rash, short stature, delayed puberty)
    ☐ developmental delay (general, language, immaturity, school failure)
    ☐ behavioural problems (attachment disorder, aggression, indiscriminate friendliness, soiling, promiscuity, truancy, stealing)
▷ sexual
  ▶ involves forcing or enticing child or young person to take part in sexual activities, whether or not the child is aware of what is happening
  ▶ may involve physical contact, or be non-contact (watching pornographic material)
  ▶ features may include:
    ☐ physical (recurrent urinary tract infections (UTIs), vaginal bleeding, pregnancy, sexually transmitted infections (STIs), genital trauma)
    ☐ behavioural (self-harm, substance misuse, enuresis, eating disorder, hostility, low self-esteem, sexually inappropriate behaviour)
▷ neglect
  ▶ persistent failure to meet child's basic physical and psychological needs, possibly resulting in serious impairment of child's health or development
  ▶ overlaps with emotional abuse
  ▶ features may include:
    ☐ physical [failure to thrive, poor hygiene, 'deprivation hands and feet'],[7] i.e. pink swollen hands and feet more commonly found in children living in deprivation)
    ☐ school avoidance, missed appointments, poor treatment compliance.

In Scotland, a further category is recognised:

▷ non-organic failure to thrive[8,9]

▶ when child's weight for age is below the fifth percentile or crosses two major percentile lines (organic causes excluded)

▶ features may include: short stature (there is conflicting opinion about developmental delay).

Evidence from Child Protection Registers in England suggests that many children experience more than one type of abuse.

Prevalence

In 2000, the National Society for the Prevention of Cruelty to Children (NSPCC) published results of a national survey[10] of almost 3000 children and young people. Its findings were alarming:

Table 4.1 ○ *NSPCC survey findings*

Category	% positive	Projected UK (total = 12 million)
Physical	7	840,000
Emotional	6	720,000
Sexual	*4–11	up to 1.3 million
Neglect	6	720,000
Bullied at school	14–15	1.7 million
Regularly shouldering adult responsibilities	20	2.4 million

Source: Cawson P, Wattam C, Brooker S, *et al. Child Maltreatment in the United Kingdom: a study of the prevalence of child abuse and neglect* London: NSPCC, 2000.[11] Used by permission of the NSPCC.

* a number of different definitions was used.

A study of 100 GPs[11] in 2000 suggested that the average GP will see fewer than two new cases of child abuse each year (higher in urban areas, lower in rural), meaning that it is difficult for practitioners to retain their skills without both regular training and having robust systems in place to guide actions when needed.

Domestic violence and abuse

There are strong links between domestic violence and abuse of children.[12, 13] Children may be the innocent-bystander witnesses to violence, but they are more likely to be abused in an environment where there is one or more violent parents or carers.[14]

We may find it challenging to advise families in this situation: our own situation or experience may make it difficult, or we may struggle to provide care for all members of the household, including the alleged perpetrator of violence or abuse. Sometimes we may need to ask colleagues for help supporting other family members, while we continue to support the victims of violence.

Vulnerable children and families

Evidence suggests that children and families move in and out of periods of higher and lower risk of abuse and neglect.[15] Children are at higher risk during times when one parent is away or ill, when financial pressures dominate, or when parents are substance misusers or offenders. However, it is also known that interventions by professionals may help to move these children and young people back into lower-risk situations. Help with benefits, housing and family support may all improve the outcomes of children in need.

The consultation

All of us working in primary care recognise the difficulty we feel in those rare consultations where we suspect that a child may be the victim of abuse. Because it happens infrequently we feel uncertain about our role. It might be helpful to have a set of policies and procedures in place that have been the subject of training and discussion within the practice. The Royal College of General Practitioners (RCGP), in collaboration with the NSPCC, has produced a Toolkit that guides practices through this process.[5]

Recording a good history is important: this may come from parents or carers, and might also include noting what the child has said (appropriate to the level of understanding). As with all difficult situations, noting actual phrases may be useful. It is relatively unusual for children to make false accusations, so we should respond appropriately to any disclosure.

Most GPs would undertake an appropriate external examination, but not of intimate areas. The signs to look for are listed above. If necessary, examination of the genitalia might be undertaken by an experienced doctor, such as a paediatrician with an interest in child protection.

Recording

Recording this information, both the history and the examination, is an area where GPs have been criticised in the past: it is helpful to make clear, contemporaneous records, with body maps where available. Read codes should be used where possible: these vary between computer systems, but codes such as 13IM (child on Protection Register) or 13IF (child at risk) should be used until Connecting for Health updates and standardises codes across systems and jurisdictions.

Unless you are familiar with guidance on recording body images, and gaining consent for their usage and distribution, you should not take photographs. If appropriate, this will be done later.

Confidentiality

Most GPs struggle to know how much of what is learned in a consultation can be shared with colleagues, particularly in other agencies. The General Medical Council offers guidance on confidentiality,[16] reinforcing the absolute duty to share information where it is:

▷ necessary to make a child or young person safe
▷ in the public interest
▷ the subject of an order of a court.

However, that still leaves questions about the duty of confidentiality due to other family members, particularly when comprehensive documents, such as minutes of child protection proceedings, may contain very personal details of other people for whom GPs also provide care. The GP is responsible for ensuring that any disclosure of information is justified by the risk to a child or young person, that it is proportionate to the situation, and that the reasons for disclosure or non-disclosure are well-recorded. Guidance on this may be sought from the UK Defence Organisations.[17]

Safeguarding processes [18-20]

Child Protection Plans

If GPs have concerns about a child, it may help to share those concerns with a practice colleague, and to see if other agencies working with the child, including health visitors, school nurses or education, share those concerns. *ContactPoint* is an England-wide service that allows professionals to find out who else is working with an individual child. It is helpful to check if the child has a Protection Plan: previously called 'checking the Child Protection Register'. This information is useful to all agencies in shaping assessment of risk. Each area service has a dedicated telephone number.

You may also consider discussing the situation with a named doctor or nurse. Each PCT must employ someone to advise professionals when to take action and what to do. Their contact details should be circulated regularly by the primary care trust.

Referral

Having recognised signs that might raise concern about abuse or neglect (and the GP does not make a diagnosis here: he or she merely acts on those concerns), it is vitally important that the practitioner responds appropriately.

If there is concern that the danger may still be present, urgent action is required to make the child safe. If not, then action may be considered and discussed with colleagues from the practice, or other agencies.

URGENT ACTION

Children's Social Care Services (CSCS) is the key agency in safeguarding. It may respond jointly with the police. Practitioners may find it helpful to have important telephone numbers listed in a directory, accessible to all team members. CSCS may use a central number as access portal at all times, or a separate number to call in or out of office hours. Telephone referral, made immediately, should be followed up by the GP in writing within 48 hours. At the end of the telephone call it should be clear to the practitioner what is going to happen and when.

NON-URGENT ACTION

Provided the child is safe, it may be appropriate to wait until normal office hours before contacting CSCS. Initial telephone contact with CSCS is best followed up by written referral within 48 hours; receipt of referral should be acknowledged within 1 working day. If GPs have not had confirmation within 3 working days, the CSCS should be contacted again.

REFERRAL FORM

Working Together to Safeguard Children recommends the use of the Common Assessment Framework Tool,[18] which allows the assessment of the child in a more rounded, three-dimensional way, considering factors relating to the child, the parents and the environment. This is the common language of all the agencies tasked with safeguarding children. A GP may only have access to certain pieces of information and not see the complete picture: other agencies may be able to complete the picture at a later stage.

SPEED OF RESPONSE

GPs sometimes feel frustrated that CSCS does not seem to respond within the usual primary care timeframe. The parameters for the response in *Working Together to Safeguard Children* call for an initial assessment to occur within 7 working days of referral.

Working with families

UK general practice is characterised by the enduring relationship between doctor, patient and family.[21] The continuation of this relationship is of importance to GPs, even after disclosure of abuse of a child. Families value honesty above most other qualities, and may often prefer to be kept informed than excluded from decisions concerning their children. Other members of the practice may provide valuable assistance by tending to the needs of other family members at a time of strain.

Working with other agencies

The structures of medical training create very different professionals from those in other agencies. We only understand one another by working together. Multi-agency training is helpful in forging shared understanding between professionals dealing with children,[22] but the benefit of such training may sometimes be offset by high staff turnover. The move towards children's centres, bringing non-health agencies together, may fracture inter-agency working for a child.

Child protection conferences

Following the initial assessment of a child in need, it may be decided that no further action is necessary, or that professionals need to share information in a case conference. Here, professionals from all agencies dealing with a child – education, CSCS, police and probation, paediatrician, health visitor, school nurse and GP – meet to share information and assess the risk to a child. This assessment may form the basis of a plan to keep the child safe. Parents and carers often attend these meetings to put their point of view.

Evidence from research[23] suggests that GPs may be reluctant to attend such meetings, but it is hugely important that they do. No other agency has access to such a breadth of information about a child and family, or the ability to make clear judgements on the basis of that information. The presence of a GP is extremely valuable to the conference.

53

Summary

Children represent many of the most vulnerable members of our society. It can be difficult for the GP to hear the child's voice among the clamour of others. Abuse and neglect are prevalent in society, and it is likely that children who are victims of abuse will also be seen by members of the GP team. We all need some level of training in recognising abuse, and to be watchful and ready for the rare occasions in which it is presented to us in our work.

Thinking it through

Take a moment to reflect on whether your practice has:

▷ an individual identified as lead for safeguarding or child protection
▷ an accessible list of important telephone numbers
▷ regular meetings to review children in need
▷ training available for all staff.

What barriers do you think prevent the practice from safeguarding children? Are your practice services children- and young person-friendly? Are your practice staff confident in their role when a child is at risk? Is the practice confident that it has systems in place to follow up children in need?

Case discussion

▶ Jane is a 3-year-old girl who has been brought by her mother because of bruising on her arms. She is said to have fallen from a playground slide 2 days before. Her mother describes her as 'hyperactive'.

▷ *What further information are you going to ask and look for?*

▶ Jane's GP record reveals three Accident and Emergency (A&E) attendances in the previous 6 months, with computer-generated letters diagnosing 'STI Lt elbow', 'Fall ?injury' and 'Head injury'.

▷ *What issues arise from the use of computer-generated correspondence?*

▶ You examine Jane, and notice a series of oval bruises on both the front and back of her upper arms. They seem to be in the shape of fingertips.

▷ *What further examination would you want to carry out?*

▶ By undressing her down to her underwear, with a chaperone present, you can see bruises of varying colours from the scapular tip down to the iliac crest on both sides, spared in the midline, with dark/light parts horizontally through them. She has bruising of the ear and inside the mouth. She has a small subconjunctival haemorrhage in the right eye.

▷ *How are you going to record these findings?*

▶ Having used the Body Maps within your computer system (e.g. Systm-One) to record these injuries, you decide to refer Jane for further assessment. At this stage, you do not know how these injuries have occurred, but you have concerns that they may not be accidental, may represent serious illness, and that Jane is certainly not safe. You therefore decide to take urgent action.

▷ *What three things are you going to do next?*

▶ You may want to share some of your concerns with the family; this is difficult. You may wish to use phrases like: 'At this point, we don't know what the cause of these bruises are', 'Now that I've examined her, I can see that there's much more going on than just the arm bruises', or 'We'll need to do further tests to find out why she has been injured in this way'. You may wish to explain that information may need to be shared with others, in Jane's best interests.

You may want to check to see what other agencies are involved (Contact-Point, England) and whether she is subject to a Protection Plan.

You may want to discuss things with a colleague in the practice, or with a named professional colleague.

▷ *Who are you going to contact to refer this child for further assessment?*

▶ It is tempting to refer this child immediately to A&E for assessment. All this achieves is to move the child out of your department and into another; it will be equally difficult for A&E to deal with, and this will not usually be in the child's best interests. There is also the uncertainty about whether or not the child will actually arrive there. Equally, we find it professionally easier to refer to a paediatrician; again, this merely shifts the child to a different department, albeit a more appropriate one.

The best course of action is usually to contact CSCS on its emergency number. The social worker may well phone you back (to verify the location of your call). You would expect immediate action within minutes, possibly a social worker coming to the surgery to take the child to hospital, or arrangements for the social worker to rendezvous with the family at the hospital. Sometimes, the involvement of a social worker may be a facilitative thing, if perhaps the family have transport difficulty and the hospital is not easily accessible.

The social worker comes to the surgery, and takes Jane and her mother to hospital. The social worker will also take a letter from you in which you summarise her medical and developmental history, immunisations and allergies. The letter should also describe her injuries and mention your concern about the fingertip pattern bruising, the bruising of varying colour or age on the back, the suggestion of toolmark bruising, and the subconjunctival haemorrhage (which may be suggestive of shaking).

A few days later, you hear from the health visitor involved with the family that a joint investigation is being carried out (England and Wales – Section 47 Children Act 2004; Section 53 The Children (Scotland) Act 1995; Article 66 The Children (NI) Order 1995). Jane is still in hospital, where a CT scan has confirmed intracranial bleeding, and a skeletal survey has shown old, healed rib fractures. It is thought that the bruising on her back has been caused by being hit with a belt. An initial child protection conference is planned for later this week.

▷ *What issues arise from attendance at case conferences?*

Convenience ▷ many GPs say that conferences are held at times and in places that are not convenient for them. There is evidence to suggest that when location and timing are changed to suit the GP, attendance is not significantly improved.

Cost ▷ most GPs feel that patients simply wait until their return from the conference and that locum doctors are expensive and do not replace them adequately. Many GPs feel that it costs the practice more to employ a locum to backfill than can be raised from the fee payable under the Collaborative Arrangements (1974). It is worth knowing that the fees charged for this service are decided by the practice, not the primary care organisation. Each practice should be calculating how much it costs to backfill a doctor, and charge appropriately.

Experience ▷ many GPs feel they lack the familiarity and experience needed to contribute to a conference. In reality, the conference is considering information with a strong medical theme, ranging from trauma and emergency care, to mental health and neurodevelopmental medicine. No other branch of medical practice has a sufficiently wide range of expertise to cover these areas.

Web resources

▷ Doctors.net. *Child Protection* (eCME module),
   **www.doctors.net.uk/ecme/wfrmIntro.aspx?groupid=40&modu
   leid=525&orgnid=3**   [log-in required].
▷ Primary Care Child Safeguarding Forum. **www.pccsf.co.uk**
   [accessed August 2009].
▷ Royal College of General Practitioners, National Society for the
   Prevention of Cruelty to Children. *Safeguarding Children and Young People
   in General Practice: a toolkit*. London: RCGP, 2008,
   **www.rcgp.org.uk/PDF/CIR_Toolkit%20document%20final
   %20edit.pdf** [accessed August 2009].
▷ General Medical Council. *0–18 years: guidance for all doctors* London:
   GMC, 2007, **www.gmc-uk.org/guidance/ethical_guidance/
   children_guidance/index.asp** [accessed August 2009].
▷ Patient UK. Growth and failure to thrive, 2007, **www.patient.co.uk/
   showdoc/40000331** [accessed August 2009].

References

1 • Royal College of General Practitioners. *Care of Children and Young People* (curriculum statement 8) London: RCGP, 2007, www.rcgp-curriculum.org.uk/pdf/curr_8_Care_of_Children_and_Young_People.pdf [accessed August 2009].

2 • Department of Health. *Practitioners with Special Interest: safeguarding children and young people* London: DoH, 2008.

3 • Department for Education and Skills. *Every Child Matters* London: TSO, 2003, www.everychildmatters.gov.uk/ [accessed August 2009].

4 • Joint Chief Inspectors Report. *Safeguarding Children: the third joint chief inspectors' report on arrangements to safeguard children* London: OFSTED, 2008, www.safeguardingchildren.org.uk/ [accessed August 2009].

5 • Royal College of General Practitioners, National Society for the Prevention of Cruelty to Children. *Safeguarding Children and Young People in General Practice: a toolkit* London: RCGP, 2008, www.rcgp.org.uk/PDF/CIR_Toolkit%20document%20final%20edit.pdf [accessed August 2009].

6 • Carter YH, Bannon MJ. *The Role of Primary Care in the Protection of Children from Abuse and Neglect* London: RCGP, 2003.

7 • Glover S, Nicoll A, Pullan C. Deprivation hands and feet *Archives of Disease in Childhood* 1985; **60**: 976–7.

8 • Boddy J, Skuse D, Andrews B. The developmental sequelae of nonorganic failure to thrive *Journal of Child Psychology and Psychiatry and Allied Disciplines* 2000; **41(8)**: 1003–14, www.ncbi.nlm.nih.gov/pubmed/11099117?dopt=Abstract [accessed August 2009].

9 • Krugman SD, Dubowitz H. Failure to thrive *American Family Physician* 2003; **68**: 5, www.aafp.org/afp/20030901/879.html [accessed August 2009].

10 • Cawson P, Wattam C, Brooker S, *et al. Child Maltreatment in the United Kingdom: a study of the prevalence of child abuse and neglect* London: NSPCC, 2000, www.nspcc.org.uk/Inform/research/Findings/childmaltreatmentintheunitedkingdom_wda48252.html [accessed August 2009].

11 • Lupton C, North N, Kahn P. What role for the general practitioner in child protection? *British Journal of General Practice* 2000; **50(461)**: 977–81, www.ingentaconnect.com/content/rcgp/bjgp/2000/00000050/00000461/art00010 [accessed August 2009].

12 • Shakespeare J, Davidson L. *Domestic Violence in Families with Children: guidance for primary health care professionals* London: RCGP, 2002, www.rcgp.org.uk/default.aspx?page=2260 [accessed August 2009].

13 • Bewley S, Friend J, Mezey G. *Violence against Women* London: RCOG Press, 1997.

14 • Abrahams C. *The Hidden Victims: children and domestic violence* London: NCH Action for Children, 1994.

15 • Cleaver H, Freeman P. *Parental Perspectives in Cases of Suspected Child Abuse* London: HMSO, 1995.

16 • General Medical Council. *0–18 years: guidance for all doctors* London: GMC, 2007, www.gmc-uk.org/guidance/ethical_guidance/children_guidance/index.asp [accessed August 2009].

17 • Medical and Dental Defence Union of Scotland. *Essential Guide to Confidentiality* Glasgow: MDDUS, 2007.

18 • Department of Health. *Working Together to Safeguard Children: a guide to inter-agency working to safeguard and promote the welfare of children* London: TSO, 2006, www.everychildmatters.gov.uk/resources-and-practice/IG00060/ [accessed August 2009].

19 • Welsh Assembly Government. *Statement on the Duties of Doctors in Investigating Child Abuse* Cardiff: WAG, 2007.

20 • The Scottish Government. *Getting it Right for Every Child* Edinburgh: TSG, 2007, www.scotland.gov.uk/Topics/People/Young-People/childrensservices/girfec [accessed August 2009].

21 • Royal College of General Practitioners. *The Future Direction of General Practice: a roadmap* London: RCGP, 2007, www.rcgp.org.uk/pdf/Roadmap_embargoed%20 11am%2013%20Sept.pdf [accessed August 2009].

22 • Carter Y, Bannon M, Limbert C, *et al.* Improving Child Protection: a systematic review of training and procedural interventions *Archives of Disease in Childhood* 2006; **91(9)**: 740–3.

23 • Polnay J C. General practitioners and child protection case conference participation *Child Abuse Review* 2000; **8**: 108–23.

Advising parents on the early years of life

5

Vince Ion

Introduction

In this chapter, we will look at some of the common issues that worry families in the early life of their newborn. Parents get information and advice from a variety of sources. This of course includes neighbours and friends, and there is a vast amount of 'folklore' about child care that can confuse and worry new parents. As healthcare professionals we need to try and adopt a consistent approach to how we support families, whilst recognising that levels of knowledge and understanding as well as health belief models and access to resources, such as the internet, vary.

As examples of some of the more common issues, the chapter will cover:

▷ birthmarks
▷ feeding difficulties
▷ sticky eye
▷ colic
▷ failure to thrive
▷ sleep disturbance
▷ constipation.

Throughout, common case histories are described to be thought over or discussed with colleagues. Not all the solutions will be found in the chapter, but the cases should provoke some discussion and this will be a good way of developing a team approach to supporting parents.

Introducing a new member to the family brings new opportunities and challenges for all family members. The issues will be different if this is a first child, where it is normal for parents to feel they do not have the skills required. For subsequent children the additional dynamic of a new baby on other children needs a different type of support.

It is worth looking again at what the RCGP curriculum specifies for excellence in the care of children and young people.

Curriculum outcomes

The competent practitioner will:[1]

▷ promote health and wellbeing by applying health promotion and disease prevention strategies appropriately, and aim to detect problems that may already be present but have not yet been detected
▷ ensure that parents or carers, children and young people receive information, advice and support to enable them to manage minor illnesses themselves
▷ prescribe and advise appropriately about the use of medicines in children and young people
▷ work effectively with colleagues across professional boundaries
▷ recognise inequalities and ethnic diversity, and address them proactively
▷ manage simultaneously both acute and chronic problems in the child, young person and family by:
  ▶ assessing children and young people's developmental needs in the context of their family and environmental factors including school and community, and parenting capacity
  ▶ understanding the key vulnerability factors for children and young people in special circumstances, and responding to their needs, including through referral and joint working
▷ referral to the health visitor and other professional for a comprehensive family needs assessment to understand and address the impact of the parent's needs on the children's health and development.

Birthmarks

A birthmark (naevus) is a coloured mark that forms on, or just below, the skin. Birthmarks are not usually hereditary; they usually develop before or shortly after birth.

Birthmarks that appear on the outside layer of the skin are known as epithelial naevi, and ones that appear on the deeper layers are known as dermal or subcutaneous naevi. The common types of birthmark include the following.

Port-wine stains

These are normally quite a dark red colour and often appear on the face and neck, although they can appear anywhere on the body and are permanent.

They sometimes get thicker and darker, and form tiny red lumps underneath the skin with age. As the child gets older laser treatment can sometimes ameliorate the appearance but specialist make-up products might be needed for camouflage.

Strawberry marks

Strawberry marks (capillary haemangiomas) develop shortly after birth. They are normally quite small, although some will enlarge (sometimes quite dramatically) before shrinking and disappearing over the first few years of life. Some take up to 10 years to disappear, and might leave a lasting mark. Parents should be advised that no intervention is the preferred course of action, since treatment might scar, and the lesions often shrink or disappear altogether.

Café au lait *spots*

These birthmarks are normally tan or light brown in colour. They are flat patches that can appear anywhere on the body and are permanent. Multiple *café au lait* spots will need to be examined to exclude neurofibromatosis.

Congenital melanocytic naevi

Congenital melanocytic naevi (CMN) are made up of pigment cells. These moles are brown or black in colour and are present at birth. Normally they are small, but sometimes they can cover large areas of the body. They are permanent and need to be protected from the sun.

Stork marks

They are light pink in colour and are present at birth around the head and scalp. Most of them disappear within 2 years of birth, but if not may require laser treatment.

One in three babies are born with birthmarks, and most will not have too many problems with them. Most birthmarks appear on the head or neck. Some however are very large and dark, and are on the face, making children and their families feel concerned about their looks. Other birthmarks can cover a large part of their body, which means children avoid wearing certain clothes, or avoid activities like swimming and other sports. Problems can start if birthmarks make parents unhappy; this can lead to the child thinking it is different.

Feeding problems

Think about the following scenario

A mother comes to see you with a new baby and a toddler. She says she is considering stopping breastfeeding the baby as she is very uncomfortable and her first child gets very upset when she breastfeeds the baby.

What are your priorities for this family and who else in the primary care team would you refer to and consult?

There is a variety of ways in which breastfeeding problems present. New mothers take a while to get the hang of breastfeeding and may worry they are not producing sufficient milk or their baby is not satisfied. However, as long as the baby is gaining weight at the normal rate, there is no need for concern. Working with, initially, the midwife and, then, the health visitor as a team usually enables families to feel well supported. Minor infections, such as a cold, can interrupt established feeding patterns, but rarely for long.[2]

The symptoms of feeding disorders can vary, but common symptoms include:

▷ colic
▷ failing to gain weight normally
▷ crying before or after food
▷ regurgitating or vomiting
▷ diarrhoea
▷ constipation
▷ refusing food
▷ lack of appetite
▷ abdominal pain
▷ behavioural problems.

Occasionally early feeding problems can be caused by anatomical problems (such as oesophageal atresia or a severe cleft palate) or less specific illness. Fortunately, fast identification is normal in these cases. Gastro-oesophageal reflux disease (GORD) can also cause problems with feeding. GORD can affect weight gain and be a source of great stress for parents.

GPs must be aware of the more serious conditions that can interfere with food absorption and weight gain. These include:

▷ food intolerance
▷ inflammatory bowel disease
▷ coeliac disease
▷ cystic fibrosis.

Emotional and social issues can be a source of feeding problems in toddlers and older children. Eating disorders such as bulimia or anorexia nervosa are more likely to develop in older children, especially girls. Feeding problems are common throughout childhood and affect both boys and girls.

What is the treatment?

The key investigation is the height and weight charts. It is a reassuring sign if the child is maintaining its position on the centiles. Expectations about what is a normal diet can vary widely, and parents faced with advice from well-meaning friends can become very concerned about patterns that are in fact not affecting health. Many feeding problems, especially in small babies, sort themselves out without the cause ever being established.

With older children, families can often make food an issue by the way in which they respond. Advice should be given to be as flexible as they can in adapting to the eating habits that suit the child. For a child described as a 'fussy eater', suggest trying a wide range of foods, perhaps in more frequent and smaller meals. The emphasis should be on health rather than weight gain. Midwives, health visitors and local support groups can be a great source of advice for parents worried about feeding problems.

Consider working with the primary care team on the following

A young single mother appears in your surgery with her own mother. She looks worried, tired and tearful, and explains that she has tried breastfeeding but cannot satisfy her baby. She asks if she should give her baby a bottle as her mum is suggesting. She also says that her breasts are uncomfortable, and although she wants to keep up with breastfeeding thinks she may have to stop. What action/advice would you suggest in such circumstances?

Sticky eye

This is most common in newborns during the first 24 hours after birth. Babies can pick up the bacteria causing sticky eye during delivery. It should be noted also that the relative shape of the baby's head may affect efficient drainage via the lacrimal duct and cause an appearance of infection.

Cleaning the baby's eyes regularly, with gentle massage over the inner canthus to stimulate tear flow, should clear it up in a day or so.

In older babies and children, a sticky and red bloodshot eye is likely to be caused by conjunctivitis, especially if bilateral.

63

Advice to help clear this condition

▷ Bathe the affected eye with cooled, boiled water.

▷ Use a clean piece of cotton wool for bathing each eye and wipe from the inner eyelid outwards.

▷ Keep a separate towel and flannel for the baby in case the discharge is being caused by an infection.

▷ If both eyes are, or become, infected or the condition does not clear up in a few days, further consultation with one of the primary care team is advised.

Conjunctivitis in an infant aged less than 1 month old is a notifiable disease in the UK. This type of conjunctivitis (ophthalmia neonatorum) may be due to an intrapartum infection and may include gonococcal or chlamydial infection.

Infantile colic

'Colic' is a word used variously by parents and others, and generally means excess crying, thought to be due to tummy ache. Babies who have colic are not ill, but they cry a lot more than other babies. The pattern includes:

▷ the baby suddenly starts a high-pitched crying and nothing that the parent does seems to help

▷ the crying can last for minutes or much longer

▷ the crying begins at the same time, often in the afternoon or evening

▷ the baby's face might become pink/red

▷ the baby draws up its legs when crying, and its tummy might look swollen

▷ the baby might make a tight fist with either or both hands.

Colic usually starts when a baby is a few weeks old and usually stops at 4 or 5 months. It is not associated with pathology and there is no effective treatment – although, naturally for such a distressing event, there are many suggested remedies.

Researchers have a variety of views as to the cause: some think that colic could be caused by wind or painful bowel cramps. Some babies might be sensitive to lactose or to protein in cow's milk. It also might be due to the development of the Peyer's patches in the gut. Other researchers think that colic is not caused by stomach problems; they think that some babies just cry a lot and some parents are more worried by their baby's crying.

Some of the triggers for colic are thought to include:

▷ maternal diet if breastfeeding – chocolate, dairy products, spicy food, caffeine, and some fruits and vegetables may all bring on colic
▷ medication that the mother might be taking that goes through to the breast milk
▷ fast feeding, especially by bottle – if the baby feeds very quickly, the hole in the bottle's teat might be too large
▷ worrying or feeling anxious about the baby.

What treatments work?

No single treatment for colic has been shown to work for sure. Here are some suggestions for families to try themselves:

▷ baby massage – there are classes to learn how to do this. One small study found that massage seemed to have an effect. As long as it is gentle, side effects seem unlikely
▷ carry the baby around more to try to comfort it; some try driving around in the car to soothe their baby
▷ some parents use the noise of a range of items, which may distract the baby
▷ moving a baby into a new room or environment may help
▷ if a baby is bottle feeding, you can also buy special teats that are designed to stop air getting into the feed
▷ if the baby is bottle fed, switching to a formula containing whey hydrolysate might help. Whey hydrolysate milk has been treated to avoid an allergic reaction in babies. However, any change in diet should be a last report as parents can get into a vicious circle of anxiety surrounding changes to the milk
▷ cranial osteopathy uses gentle pressure on the bones of the cranium and purports to help with colic. There has not been any significant research in this area.

How to advise families to cope with colic

When a baby has colic, family life is turned upside down. It is extremely stressful and upsetting when a baby cries for hours and cannot be comforted. For first-time parents in particular it can be a shock to discover that a new-born baby appears to be in distress and will not settle to sleep. They may feel guilty and anxiety levels will mount. Colic does not harm a baby's development – in fact, children with colic are actually very stimulated! However, saying this to a parent is unlikely to relieve the stress caused by the crying.

Suggest that parents take turns in comforting the baby, so that one can rest while the other is awake. Family, friends and support groups can be helpful as reinforcement and can reduce the pressure on parents. Encourage parents to ask for help, rather than finding themselves over-tired and stressed, and to talk to other parents who have experienced the same thing. The health visitor can usually put them in touch with others who have experienced this condition. Finally, do not forget to remind parents that colic is only temporary.

Think about the following scenario

A grandmother approaches the health visitor saying she is concerned that her daughter and son-in-law are becoming depressed, as their baby is constantly crying. They have been advised by friends to try gripe water and other home-made remedies. How would you address this?

What approach would you discuss with other members of the primary healthcare team to support this family?

Failure to thrive

Failure to thrive is a description applied to children whose current weight or rate of weight gain is significantly below that of other children of similar age and sex.[3]

Assessment

When assessing growth in all children, both height and weight should be considered, and, in small children, head circumference as well. The height and weight should be on roughly the same centiles. To diagnose failure to thrive it is imperative to understand normal growth and variation. For example, it is normal for a baby to lose up to 10 per cent of body weight in the first few days of life. This is rapidly regained but more slowly in breastfed babies. The health visitor working within the primary healthcare team will assess this routinely and will have access, as we all do, to the centile charts within the child health record.

There are separate centile charts for boys and girls as the former tend to be bigger. There may well be some racial differences too. Children of Asian background are often a little smaller. Look at the parents: tall parents have tall children and short parents have short children. The genetic component of height and weight tends to become manifest between birth and 2 years of age. Hence children of small parents may cross the centiles at this age. About 25 per cent of normal children will shift to a lower centile line in the first 2 years of life. If there are small parents and a healthy, happy child, there is no cause for concern.[4]

Look at the charts but do not forget to look at the child!

Can failure to thrive be treated?

Watching mothers as they breastfeed or bottle feed is essential. Is the baby's jaw working correctly or is the baby having trouble sucking? Thrush is a common cause for feeding problems in the early days and weeks of life.

The treatment could be a matter of simply breast/bottle feeding the baby more often to increase the baby's food intake. Mothers who want to continue to breastfeed should avoid the temptation to 'top up' feeds with formula milk. Breastfeeding is a finely balanced physiological activity and it is the baby's suckling that stimulates milk production. A baby full up on bottled feeds will not suck for so long and the breast production will reduce. Also the action needed for breastfeeding is very different from feeding from a bottle and, especially early on, bottle feeding may interfere with development of a good feeding action in a mixed-feed baby.

Prevention

▷ Good antenatal care and avoidance of recreational drugs, tobacco and alcohol in pregnancy (although there is some current debate on this) will reduce the risk.

▷ Parenting classes will lead to a better understanding of the needs of the baby. Nowadays fathers are often involved too and this is to be welcomed.

▷ An astute midwife or health visitor should detect problems before they become serious.[5]

If feeding difficulties are excluded and serial weights show the child is losing or not gaining weight then referral for further investigation should be made.

Behavioural problems

Behavioural problems can occur in children of all ages. Toddlers and young children may refuse to do as they are asked by adults. They can appear to be rude and have tantrums. Hitting and kicking of other people is common. So is breaking or spoiling things that matter to others.

Accentuate the positive

For parents, especially in today's busy lifestyle where by necessity both parents may need to work, it can be easy not to notice children when they are being good, and only pay attention to them when they are behaving badly. If children in busy households only get attention when they are breaking rules, they may continue with that behaviour to gain parental attention. Most children, including teenagers, need and want the attention from their parents, and will do whatever it takes to get it. It is easy to see how, over time, a 'vicious cycle' can develop.

Most child development from a psycho-social perspective can be learnt. Encouraging parents to acknowledge good behaviour and at the early stages at least ignore bad behaviour is a good starting point. If bad behaviour gets to a point where it cannot be ignored it is important that we support the family and encourage them to continue responding more favourably to good behaviour than bad.[6]

More serious problems

Some children have more serious behavioural problems. Some of the indications are:

▷ if the child continues to behave badly for a number of weeks/months, and is repeatedly being disobedient, cheeky, aggressive or even violent
▷ if the behaviour is out of the ordinary or breaks the rules that a family is unhappy about.

This can become much more than ordinary childish mischief or adolescent rebelliousness, can affect a child's development, and can interfere with its ability to lead a normal life.[7] Serious behavioural problems can be extremely disruptive for both the child and the family. This kind of behaviour puts a huge strain on the family.

Children who have serious behavioural problems will often find it difficult to make friends. They may be bright or in the normal range but they do not do well at school. The young person may be feeling that he or she cannot do anything right. He or she often blames others including family members for his or her difficulties and will not know how to change.

How can we help?

It helps if discipline is fair and consistent, and it is crucial for both parents to agree on how to handle their child's behaviour. All children want the praise and rewards from their families when the behaviour improves. Praise even for the small everyday things is very effective. It lets the child know that the parents love and appreciate him or her.

If the behaviour has also extended to school it is helpful if parents and teachers can work together. The extended team should, and can, often help when advice is sought from teachers, a school nurse or from an educational psychologist.

If more specialist help is needed, a referral to the Child and Adolescent Mental Health Services (CAMHS) might be indicated. Specialists can help by finding out what is causing the problem, and also by suggesting practical ways of improving the difficult behaviour.

69

Sleep disturbance

Settling problems (difficulty getting off to sleep and setting down at night) and frequent night waking are experienced by about 20–30 per cent of children aged 1–5 years. These sleep problems often continue into toddlerhood. A second peak in sleep problems occurs in teenagers, where sleep-timing problems can cause family discord and include delayed sleep due to lifestyle issues. Such children have difficulty getting off to sleep, and then problems getting up in the morning for school.

Sleep problems can be divided into two broad areas: abnormalities of sleep activity (parasomnias) and abnormalities of sleep patterns (dysomnias). This latter is what families are most concerned about in early life due to the disruption it can cause.

Parasomnias

These are often caused by inappropriately timed activation of physiological systems. They include nightmares, sleep terrors and sleepwalking. There is no specific intervention that will help with these and the child will often grow out of them. Parents should be advised to maintain a safe environment, reassure other children who might be woken by such activity, and await peaceful sleep.

Dysomnias

These are problems that involve either excessive daytime sleepiness or difficulty initiating or staying asleep. They include: insomnia, hypersomnia, narcolepsy, breathing-related sleep disorders, and circadian rhythm sleep disorder.

Risk factors

Factors related to an increased likelihood of sleep disorders include colic, being the first born, and children with a difficult temperament. Other factors have been suggested, such as being born prematurely and low birthweight. However, evidence of such associations is contradictory. These factors may influence the onset of a sleep disorder, but the factors influencing the maintenance of a sleep problem are likely to be different.

The proportion of rapid eye movement (REM – active sleep) is higher in infants than in adults. REM is frequently associated with awakenings, and infants with a sleep disorder often need assistance to resume sleep after such arousals.

Sleep problems tend to occur more often in children with physical and learning difficulties. Pain and discomfort are obvious causes of sleep disturbance. Medications are known to cause sleep problems – such as severe drowsiness with many antiepileptic drugs.

Sleep problems can be a significant disrupter of family life and can give rise to significant stress and anxiety. As parents are up at night, trying to settle infants, they too become tired and irritable. Interventions such as advice about 'sleep hygiene' – a good bedtime routine and a consistent approach – can be very effective.

Think about the following scenario

▶ Your practice nurse reports at the primary healthcare team meeting that she has seen an experienced mother with four children who is having problems with her second child, a boy who is 6 years old.

She says this started soon after she arrived home with her newly born daughter and she is concerned about how to deal with this problem. Which members of the primary healthcare team can help with this problem and how would you suggest the team proceeds?

Constipation

Parents can mean very different things when they use the term constipation so it is worth spending some time working out exactly what is the problem.

Constipation in children presents as:

▷ difficulty when passing stools
▷ pain when passing stools
▷ passing stools less often than normal.

A mild bout of not having the bowels open in infants and children is not unusual and can last for a few days. A good diet and plenty of fluids is the best and most effective advice and treatment. Some children do develop chronic constipation, and help will be required. Chronic constipation is less common and treatment is different.[8]

What causes constipation in infants and children?

The most common reason why children become constipated is that they do not eat enough foods with fibre and they do not drink enough fluids. These are also the most common causes of constipation with adults, so it gives members of the primary healthcare team the opportunity to address not only the current problem as it presents but also deal with the lifestyle health promotion for all the family.

When children begin potty training problems can arise if the child becomes anxious and if the family approach to this is not sensitive. This can cause the child to hold the stool. The child has the feeling of needing the toilet, but resists it. The child may look uncomfortable, cross its legs, or sit on the back of the heels. With time, water is reabsorbed from the stool, which gets harder, more bulky and even more difficult to pass.

Prevention

Eating foods with plenty of fibre and taking plenty of fluids makes stools softer, larger and easy to pass. Ensuring children get enough exercise is also thought to help. A change to a high-fibre diet is often 'easier said than done', so a family approach to this lifestyle change may help.

Children are often described as fussy eaters. However, small changes in diet can and do become effective with this condition. Some examples of simple changes are:

▷ jacket potatoes with baked beans

▷ dried apricots or raisins for snacks instead of sweets
▷ porridge or other high-fibre cereals for breakfast rather than high sugar-based cereal
▷ fruit available with and between meals.

Advise parents to encourage children to drink plenty, particularly water. Squash, fizzy drinks or milk make children less likely to eat proper meals with food that contains plenty of fibre as they become 'full' more quickly with these types of fluids. In addition to water, fruit juices, such as prune, pear or apple juice, can have a laxative action, and support the fluid intake required. The amount of fluids required for both children and adults is usually underestimated, and this is usually the first line of treatment for constipation in all family members.

Treatment of chronic constipation

This commonly occurs in children between the age of 2 and 4 years. Symptoms and features include:

▷ repeated occasions when a child is uncomfortable when passing a stool
▷ the child soils regularly with soft faeces, or stained mucus. This is often described by parents as diarrhoea
▷ the child becomes upset, will not eat much, feels sick, complains of lower stomach pains and may be generally presenting as unwell.

A high-fibre diet and lots of fluids is again the first line of treatment. Laxatives are used with the aim of clearing any impacted stool. This is usually done fairly quickly with a good dose of a laxative. After the impacted stool has been cleared, it is important to continue with 'maintenance' laxative.

Top tips on child health promotion

▷ Work as a whole team.
▷ Health promotion is often a key to treatment of minor ailments.
▷ Have a lead within the practice on health promotion.
▷ Have clear objectives and priorities with regard to minor ailments.
▷ Make training available for all staff.
▷ Ensure that your practice and services are family friendly, to encourage patients to ask about the early years of life.
▷ Keep an easily accessible list of other resources available to families on early-years development and minor ailments.

▷ Have regular meetings to review the latest key issues in relation to health promotion.

Web resources

▷ Department for Children, Schools and Families, **www.dcsf.gov.uk/ index.htm** [accessed August 2009].

▷ General Medical Council. *0–18 years: guidance for all doctors* London: GMC, 2007, **www.gmc-uk.org/guidance/ethical_guidance/ children_guidance/index.asp** [accessed August 2009].

▷ MedlinePlus, **http://medlineplus.gov/** [accessed August 2009].

▷ More J. *How to Cope with Toddler Feeding Problems* Norwich: BabyCentre, 2006, **www.babycentre.co.uk/toddler/nutrition/ howtocopefeedingproblems/** [accessed August 2009].

▷ Netdoctor.co.uk, **www.netdoctor.co.uk/** [accessed August 2009].

▷ NHS Choices, **www.nhs.uk/Pages/homepage.aspx** [accessed August 2009].

73

References

1 • Royal College of General Practitioners. *Care of Children and Young People* (curriculum statement 8) London: RCGP, 2007, www.rcgp-curriculum.org.uk/pdf/curr_8_Care_of_ Children_and_Young_People.pdf [accessed August 2009].

2 • Cooper P J, Stein A. *Childhood Feeding Problems and Adolescent Eating Disorders* London: Routledge, 2006.

3 • Sherry B, Mei Z, Grummer-Strawn L. Evaluation of and recommendations for growth references for very low birth weight infants in the United States *Paediatrics* 2003; **111(4[1])**: 750–8.

4 • Krugman S D, Dubowitz H. Failure to thrive *American Family Physician* 2003; **68(5)**: 1.

5 • Ramsay M, Gisel G E, McClusker D, *et al.* Infant sucking ability, non-organic failure to thrive, maternal characteristics, and feeding practices: a prospective cohort study *Developmental Medicine and Child Neurology* 2002; **44**: 405–14.

6 • Carr A. *What Works with Children and Adolescents? A critical review of psychological interventions with children, adolescents and their families* London: Brunner-Routledge, 2000.

7 • Rutter M, Taylor E. *Child and Adolescent Psychiatry* (4th edn) London: Blackwell, 2002.

8 • Jackson P, Clayden G. *Constipation in Children: assessment and management – in association with BNF for Children* London: BMJ Learning, 2006.

Problems in the first year of life

6

Tony Choules and Mohammad Sawal

Introduction

One of the fundamental points to remember when assessing the young baby is that the body systems have not yet established or proven themselves. A systematic method of review (as used in the newborn, day 7 and 6-week checks) can help avoid obvious pitfalls when examining a child in the first year of life. As the child grows it is easier to direct examinations following a more systems-based approach, such as would be used in a toddler/older child.

This chapter considers some of the most important abnormalities that present in the first year of life. Some conditions discussed in this chapter are specific to infants while others may be discovered in later childhood.

Before reading on, consider the following self-assessment questions.

Self-assessment quiz

1 ▷ Jaundice on day 1 of life is part of the normal physiological process ▶ **True / False**.
2 ▷ Bilateral undescended testis in a newborn baby requires urgent referral ▶ **True / False**.
3 ▷ A heart murmur on day 1 of life is usually pathological ▶ **True / False**.
4 ▷ A well, breastfed baby who is gaining weight does not need investigation for jaundice at 3 weeks of age ▶ **True / False**.
5 ▷ A baby with an intermittent squint should be referred for assessment at 3 months of age ▶ **True / False**.
6 ▷ An infant with an umbilical hernia should be referred for surgical correction if it has not disappeared by 1 year of age ▶ **True / False**.

Jaundice

There are three types of neonatal jaundice classified by the age at which they present:

Jaundice on day 1 (early jaundice)

This almost invariably represents sepsis or haemolysis. The child should be referred to secondary care immediately.

Jaundice from day 2 to day 14

This may still be pathological and a general assessment is appropriate, taking into account feeding, behaviour (alert/drowsy), perfusion, urine output, etc. However, most jaundice in this period will be physiological (normal haemolysis, resolution of bruising and 'sluggish' hepatic function). Even in the well baby high levels of bilirubin (generally considered to be > 300 micromol/l in the term baby) require phototherapy, and referral for assessment may be appropriate. The unwell baby should be referred immediately. If the baby is well and the bilirubin level below the cut-off for treatment then reassurance may be given. Daily review by the midwife may be required.

Jaundice after day 14 (prolonged jaundice)

Any jaundice lasting beyond 2 weeks of age is 'prolonged' and requires investigation. Most cases in breastfed babies will be 'breast milk jaundice' and, if the tests suggest this, then reassurance may be given along with the advice that the jaundice may persist as long as breastfeeding continues. A few babies will have a pathological cause including biliary obstruction, which shows up on testing as a conjugated hyperbilirubinaemia. This rare but significant condition is amenable to surgical correction if done in the first 2 months of life. Unfortunately clinical examination is almost completely unhelpful in differentiating pathological prolonged jaundice from benign causes, so referral for investigation within a few days of presentation with prolonged jaundice is mandatory.

Heart murmurs

Significant congenital heart disease is often detected antenatally. If not, it will usually present within the first few days of life with cardiac failure, cyanosis and/or shock. Most heart murmurs detected on routine examination thus almost always represent minor abnormalities at worst, although some will require monitoring and possibly surgical correction.

If a murmur is detected a full cardiovascular examination should be undertaken including colour (preferably oxygen saturations), perfusion, the presence of femoral pulses and signs of cardiac failure (hepatomegaly and/ or respiratory distress).

Common pathological heart murmurs are listed in Table 6.1.

Many newborn babies will have a heart murmur in the first few days of life. Heart murmurs that do not have a pathological cause will disappear, and the well infant can be reviewed at 24 or 48 hours of age. Other non-pathological (innocent) murmurs are normal sounds made by the heart that are probably more easily heard in children because of a more rapid heart rate and thinner chest wall.

Table 6.1 ○ **Summary of characteristics of common paediatric heart murmurs**

Lesion	Murmur	Location	Radiation	Heart Sounds	Notes
VSD	Pansystolic Harsh	LLSB (4LICS)	—	Normal though S2 may be obscured	Large VSDs may not give rise to a murmur as there is no pressure gradient between the ventricles
PS	ES	ULSB (2LICS)	Lung fields	Wide variable split S2	May radiate to the back
PDA	Continuous	ULSB (infra-clavicular)	Also heard between shoulder blades	Normal – gallop may be present if large flow	
ASD	ES	ULSB (2LICS)		Fixed split S2	
AS	ES	URSB (2RICS)	Neck	Narrow split S2	
(Stills)	Musical	LLSB (3LICS)		Normal	Intensity of these murmurs varies with posture (listen lying and sitting)
Venous hum	Continuous hum	URSB and supra-clavicular		Normal	Disappears with pressure over the neck/ shoulder

Key: **AS** = aortic stenosis, **ASD** = atrial septal defect, **ES** = ejection systolic, **LLSB** = lower left sternal border, **L/RICS** = left/right intercostal space (approximate location in 'classical' murmurs), **PDA** = patent ductus arteriosus, **PS** = pulmonary stenosis, **ULSB** = upper left sternal border, **URSB** = upper right sternal border, **VSD** = ventricular septal defect.

Common congenital abnormalities

The list of congenital abnormalities given below is not exhaustive but includes those common abnormalities presenting in primary care.

Undescended testis (unilateral)

The incidence at birth is approximately 3 per cent (more common in premature babies) with a prevalence at 1 year of 1 per cent. They are unlikely to spontaneously descend after that, hence needing surgical correction (orchidopexy) at approximately 1 year of age. Undescended testes have an increased risk of malignancy and reduced sperm production. These risks are thought to be reduced by surgery. Men with a single testis will have a reduced sperm count but the effect on fertility is not usually significant. Examine from the inguinal ring, trying to draw the testis down into the scrotum, being aware of highly retractile testes that can retract to the level of the inguinal ring, especially in the cold.

Undescended testis (bilateral)

If it is not possible to find both testes, examine the genitalia carefully and consider the possibility of an intersex condition. Refer to secondary care (urgently if within the first few days of life, because of the association with electrolyte imbalance). Intersex is much less likely if one or both testes are palpable.

Pre-auricular skin tags

These are present in up to 1 per cent of newborn babies and are usually of no significance. Some studies have suggested association with hearing and renal abnormalities. They may be part of a number of congenital malformations (syndromes), in which case other features may be found. Parental pressure may require a referral for surgery for cosmetic reasons.

Hypospadias

This results from incomplete development of the urethra. Severity ranges from mild abnormalities of the foreskin to a urethral opening at the base of the penis. In severe cases intersex conditions must be considered (see 'undescended testis' above). Surgical correction is usually required and advice should be given against circumcision as the foreskin is used for the reconstruction.

'Dislocated' hips

Developmental dysplasia of the hips (DDH) covers dislocated and dislocat-able hips. The Barlow–Ortolani manœuvre should be used to abduct the hips and feel for relocation of a dislocated hip, as well as fixing the pelvis and pushing to dislocate a dislocatable hip – subsequent abduction may then relocate it. This is represented diagrammatically in Chapter 2.

Positive tests are usually felt as a 'clunk' rather than a 'click'. Clicks are usually ligamentous and probably of no significance. Babies with positive tests should be referred to secondary care (usually orthopaedics or paedi-atrics). Parents should be told to apply 'double nappies' (a second nappy around the usual one to increase abduction and therefore stabilise a dislo-catable joint). A baby with an equivocal test may warrant an ultrasound. In such a case double nappies should also be recommended as this may help to resolve a minor instability. Risk factors for DDH include family history, breech or other abnormal presentation, delivery by caesarean section and being female.

Accessory digits

Skin tags on the hands may be rudimentary digits. These can be removed by a plastic surgeon. The traditional management of tying off the base with cotton is generally not currently recommended.

Single palmar creases

These can be a manifestation of trisomy 21 (Down's syndrome) but are also relatively common in the general population.

Umbilical hernia

These generally resolve over the first few years of life. Occasionally surgery is carried out, although this is largely for cosmetic reasons.

Inguinal hernia

This presents as a swelling in the scrotum that may increase and decrease in size. A 'thickening' of the spermatic cord can often be felt. They always require surgical correction. Previous advice that such correction was urgent was probably not justified, but there is a risk of incarceration (failure to reduce) and/or strangulation (incarceration with compromise to the blood supply). Surgical referral should thus be timely (within a week or two) with advice to the parents to seek medical review if the hernia becomes large and fixed or appears to be causing the child distress. In such cases reduction is sometimes possible by lifting above the inguinal ring and trying to massage the hernia back through it. Sedation may ease the process.

Hydrocele

This is a collection of fluid around the testis and may be unilateral or bilateral. It may be mistaken for a hernia, but a hydrocele will transilluminate and the cord will not be thickened (though with a large, tense hydrocele this latter sign may not be easy to elicit). Hydroceles almost always resolve with time.

Asymmetrical head/abnormal head shape

Asymmetry in the body is quite common. Sometimes it is more marked (e.g. hemihypertrophy). Asymmetry of the head may be part of a generalised asymmetry or occur in isolation. An abnormal head shape is usually related to posture and the plasticity of the skull. Such changes will resolve (or at least become barely noticeable) with time. Parents should be advised to position the child's head away from the flattened area in sleep where possible. Some companies produce helmets that help to correct head shape but, although measurable, the effect is probably not clinically significant in most cases. Occasionally abnormal head shape is due to craniosynostosis (premature fusion of the skull bones). This leads to a progressively abnormal head shape and requires surgical correction. It is often part of a generalised congenital syndrome. Many affected babies have obvious changes from birth. Progression rather than resolution after the first few months of life, particularly with careful positioning, should be investigated with a skull X-ray or cranial CT.

Birthmarks

Many babies have marks on the skin. A number of common birthmarks are recognised:

STORK MARKS

These are red marks on the forehead and/or nape of the neck. These are very common and will fade with time.

HAEMANGIOMAS

STRAWBERRY NAEVI

These are an intradermal and subdermal collection of dilated blood vessels. They are raised above the skin but compressible, and they grow in size over the first year of life. They then usually regress, leaving little more than a slight whorl on the skin. Strawberry naevi may bleed and ulcerate, and can become infected. They are best left alone unless complications arise (or the lesion is in a critical place – affecting vision, obstructing the nose or causing problems with eating). They can be referred for treatment with steroid injection and laser therapy.

PORT-WINE STAIN

This is an intradermal haemangioma (largely venous). It is not raised but is disfiguring. It does not lead to other complications but can be referred for treatment with steroid injection and laser therapy.

('MONGOLIAN') BLUE SPOT

This is usually found at the base of the spine. It is very common in babies with dark skin but can also present in Caucasians. It may be confused with bruising and lead to false allegations of physical abuse. It is important to document.

BIRTHMARKS OVER THE SPINE/SACRAL PITS

These may indicate subtle spinal cord malformations, including spina bifida occulta and cord tethering. Haemangiomas or simple sacral pits (in which the base can be seen and are no more than 2.5 cm from the anus) are unlikely to cause a problem but hairy patches or abnormal skin folds may be more significant. Spinal ultrasound may exclude most problems in the newborn. Beyond this age an MRI may be necessary.

Finger/toe syndactyly

Joining or webbing of the digits can occur in the toes or the fingers. Toe syndactyly (usually second or third) is rarely a problem but may be part of an underlying syndrome. Finger syndactyly will require plastic surgery review.

Squints (strabismus)

These should be referred to ophthalmology if persistent at 6 months.

Sticky/watery eyes

In some babies development of the tear ducts can be completed after birth. These babies frequently have watery eyes that can be 'sticky' after periods of sleep. The only treatment required is gentle cleaning with cool, boiled water. Antibiotic ointment is only required for clear evidence of infection/inflammation.

Child development in the first year

In general practice childhood developmental assessment is part of the Child Health Promotion Programme. Being able to assess children for developmental difficulties is very important as it enables early referral for diagnosis and intervention (medical, environmental and educational).

▶ The parents of an 11-month-old baby bring her to see you. They are worried because she is not sitting. When supported on her mother's lap she seems happy, though is wary of you when you approach her. She is making recognisable sounds, 'dada', 'baba', etc. She reaches for objects offered to her and takes hold of them in a simple pincer grasp. She then regards them and easily passes them from hand to hand.

▷ *Should you reassure the parents or refer?*

Normal child development

The normal development follows a recognised sequence in most children and this can be affected by a variety of factors (Table 6.2).

Table 6.2 ○ *Factors affecting child development*

Prenatal	Intrapartum	Postnatal
Foetal		
Chromosomal	Problems in labour, e.g. cord prolapse, shoulder dystocia	Social problems, e.g. social deprivation, neglect
Genetic, e.g. metabolic		Environmental factors, e.g. toxins
		Cultural factors
		Nutrition
Maternal		
Infection, e.g. TORCH		
Alcohol/drug use		
Nutrition		
Chronic disease		

Children acquire different skills at different ages and always move from one skill to the next. There is a significant variation of the normal range. For defining the range of normal for each milestone the median age is used, which means that 50 per cent of children are expected to achieve the skill at a particular age.

Sometimes it can be more useful to know the 25th or 95th centile (e.g. 25 per cent of children will be sitting at 6 months and 95 per cent by 11 months); if the skill has not been achieved by this age, it is likely to be of concern. An individual child may show a slight variation in skill level in different areas of development (e.g. some children are more advanced in gross motor skills and less advanced in speech and language skills or vice versa). It is important to recognise abnormal or delayed development and refer for assessment as appropriate. Loss of skills is particularly concerning and should warrant swift referral to identify any potentially treatable (e.g. metabolic) condition.

Categories of development

The developmental skills can be categorised in the following four areas:

▷ gross motor
▷ fine motor and vision
▷ speech language and hearing
▷ social.

A summary of skills acquired over the first year is given in Table 6.3 (p. 86).

GROSS MOTOR

The rate of development within this area varies depending upon the state of child health, the degree of stimulation and even surroundings. Children follow different patterns of events that lead to walking, including crawling, creeping and bottom shuffling. Those who bottom shuffle are usually late to walk because it is more difficult to get to the upright posture from the sitting position. Some children go straight from sitting to walking without any intervening stage.

Part of the motor development is the suppression of primitive reflexes (e.g. Moro, asymmetric tonic neck reflexes). Children with cerebral palsy frequently exhibit these primitive reflexes at an age when they would have disappeared in children with normal development. Global developmental problems usually present with motor problems initially because these are earlier and more recognisable milestones. It is important to try to distinguish these from purely motor problems, e.g. those due to muscular weakness.

FINE MOTOR SKILLS AND VISION

Fine motor skills depend upon normal vision and appropriate opportunity for learning. They are very much closely linked together. Acuity at birth is around 6/120 and develops rapidly so that large objects (e.g. faces) will be regarded by 2 to 3 weeks of age, then followed in a 180 degree arc by 2 to 3 months. At 1 year acuity is about 6/18. In the first few months of life, visual abilities begin to integrate with hand skills such as reaching for the object (ulnar approach, radial approach and, finally, direct approach), grabbing the object in the hand (palmar grasp evolving to simple pincer and then fine pincer) and transferring from one hand to the other. Subsequently, the infant develops the ability to focus on rapidly moving objects; during the second year the child develops an interest in pictures, and the hand skills become more refined. Visual and co-ordination/muscular problems will clearly cause problems in this area of development.

Speech and language and hearing

Speech and language development can be divided into two fields:

▷ pre-lingual and receptive
▷ expressive language (vocalisation).

Vocalisation starts as an open, wobble sound ('cooing'). This is followed by 'babble,' which soon begins to contain recognisable sounds from the native language.

In the first 2 years of life, receptive language develops from recognition of single words to the ability to recognise and label objects and pictures. This is closely followed by expressive language development of those labels (usually single words but sometimes a 'label' may be more than one word, e.g. 'Granddad Paul' is a single label). Single labels are then joined into two word phrases and then more complex sentences. Children also use different gestures, particularly pointing to request (from about 1 year) and to show object of interest, which is a major part of their nonverbal communication.

Hearing problems are the commonest cause of delay in this area of development. Refer any child with such a delay for a hearing test. Behavioural problems may present initially as language delay.

Social and behaviour

Social development in the same way goes through different phases. At the age of 6 weeks, the first social interaction children make is to start smiling when spoken to. The further progress is to respond to obvious friendly handling by the age of 3 months and then reaching for an object to putting it in their mouth by 6 months. Older infants start holding things in their hands and chewing/taking little bites of biscuits by 9 months. They wave bye-bye as a friendly gesture by 12 months. Towards the end of the first year children clearly distinguish known adults from strangers and behave differently towards them. All these age limits are the average and obviously there is a variation when the children achieve these developmental milestones.

Table 6.3 ○ *Summary of skills acquired over the first year of life*

	Gross motor	Fine motor and vision	Hearing, speech and language	Social and behavioural
6–8 weeks	Some head control, head to neutral in ventral suspension	Fixes on face, may follow to 90 degrees	Stills to noise	Smiles
3 months	Lifts head prone	Follows face		Hand regard
6 months	Rolling, sits unaided	Reaches for and grasps objects, palmar grasp, transfers	Cooing	Laughs, puts objects to mouth
9 months	Crawling	Radial approach with reach	Polysyllabic/ polytonal babble	Peek-a-boo, follows fallen toys
1 year	Cruising/ walking (13 months is 50th centile for walking)	Simple pincer, points (fine pincer usually by 13 months)	'Mama', 'dada' with meaning, possibly other words	Waves bye-bye, drinks from cup, points for needs, casting, shy with strangers

DEVELOPMENTAL ASSESSMENT

A number of methods are used formally for more detailed assessments. These include:

▷ Griffiths Mental Developmental Skills, 0–8 years[1]
▷ Schedule of Growing Skills, 0–5 years[2]
▷ Bayley's Scales of Infant Development, 0–42 months.[3]

In general practice informal developmental assessment can be made using parental history, a range of appropriate toys and a background knowledge of development. The Schedule of Growing Skills is widely used in primary care, but with knowledge of the child's age appropriate questions can be asked and tasks set. With experience and seeing more children, one can appreciate any significant variation between different areas of development and from that expected for the age of the child.

The general principle of assessment is to use a structured approach. Set tasks using clear language, do not leave long gaps between tasks and keep it fun. When making an assessment observe not only the completion of the task but also the quality of how the child performs. The presence of 'risk factors' (Table 6.4) should lead to consideration of referral or, perhaps, review after a period of a month or two depending on the skill assessed and age of the child. If the child shows delay in more than two areas, it is suggestive of global developmental delay and should be referred to a specialist centre (usually the local child development centre) for detailed assessment.

Table 6.4 ○ **Warning signs of developmental problems**

	Gross motor	Fine motor and vision	Hearing, speech and language	Social
6–8 weeks	Marked head lag	No fixing	No startle/ stilling to sound	No smiling
	Asymmetric reflexes			
10–12 months	Unable to sit	Hand preference	No babbling/ cooing	No differentiation of family and strangers
	Absence of saving reactions			
	Persistent primitive reflexes			

Hearing

Hearing impairment affects the social, emotional and educational development of the child. The prevalence of severe permanent congenital hearing impairment is about one per 1000. Two to three per 1000 will have moderate impairment. Early detection of hearing impairment and early intervention lessens the impact of deafness in children.

Newborn screening

By 2006 all districts in the UK had implemented a neonatal screening programme. The aim of the newborn screening is to identify all children who
have a hearing impairment. Those who do not pass the screen are referred
for more detailed diagnostic assessment. Certain 'at risk groups' (Box 6.1)
are referred for audiological review at 7 to 8 months, even if they successfully complete the screen.

The tests used by the newborn hearing screening service include:

▷ oto-acoustic emission (OAE), which provides sensitive and accurate
   means of identification of cochlear hearing impairment
▷ automated auditory brainstem response test (AABR), which provides
   accurate assessment of auditory pathways rather than cochlear
   response.

Box 6.1 ○ **Risk factors in the newborn period triggering audiology follow-up**

▷ Congenital infection.
▷ Craniofacial anomalies.
▷ Family history (first-degree relatives).
▷ Bacterial meningitis.
▷ Neonatal ventilation >5 days.
▷ Exchange transfusion.
▷ Neurodevelopmental/neurodegenerative disorders.
▷ Syndromes associated with hearing loss.

Later problems

Outside the neonatal period hearing impairment should be suspected and
an appropriate referral to audiology for hearing test arranged in the following situations:

▷ parental or professional concerns
▷ speech delay
▷ meningitis
▷ high aminoglycoside levels
▷ chronic middle-ear effusion
▷ significant head trauma
▷ neurodevelopmental disorders.

Management

Children found to have a hearing impairment are followed up by audiology services. Assessment by a multidisciplinary team including audiologist, ear, nose and throat (ENT) surgeon and teacher for the deaf is usually required. Management may include the provision of hearing aids or cochlear implants, use of signing and educational support.

Vision

Vision is the most important conduit of our learning. Children's development is highly dependent on normal vision, and more than 70 per cent of early learning is visually dependent. Visual impairment can affect language development, behaviour, fine motor skills and ultimately education and progress in school. About 7 to 8 per cent of the children leaving school have significant reduction in visual acuity although significant visual impairments are rare in the UK.

89

Visual impairment can be caused by failure of light to enter the eye (e.g. a birthmark over or around the eye, ptosis, cataracts), refractory abnormalities (myopia: near-sightedness, hypermetropia: long-sightedness and astigmatism in which there is asymmetrical focusing due to distortion), impaired ocular movement (squint/strabismus), vitreal and retinal abnormalities (e.g. retinopathy of prematurity) and neurological defects. Development of the visual pathways requires light to be focused on the retina. In conditions where light cannot reach the retina (e.g. lens opacities) or the child does not use the eye for other reasons (e.g. refractory abnormalities, strabismus) the visual pathways will not develop properly, leading to amblyopia (permanent visual loss) in that eye. In these cases early detection and treatment is vital to ensure amblyopia is prevented.

Vision testing in children is very difficult but problems should be anticipated if there is an absent red reflex on neonatal examination (absent 'green reflex' in children with more pigmented skins), family history of visual problems (squint, amblyopia and visual impairment), roving uncoordinated eye movements after 6 weeks, strabismus (a squint) present at 6 months, in children with other disabilities (e.g. cerebral palsy) and in pre-term babies who receive intensive-care therapy. Children should also be screened for visual impairment if the parents suspect a problem. Assessment should be carried out by a children's optometrist.

Management

Children with confirmed visual impairment may require multi-professional assessment and management by a team consisting of ophthalmologist, orthoptist, community child health, education, visually impaired team and social services to support children and families.

Growth problems in the first year

Growth problems in the first year of a child's life that present to the GP are usually explained by nutritional and behavioural causes. (Behaviour in this context refers to that of the parents as well as the infant.) A small proportion of infants will fail to grow because of chronic disease. Babies who are born very small for gestational age (previously referred to as 'growth retarded') often remain small despite intensive nutritional input.

It is important to remember that many babies will move from their birth centile (a reflection of maternal health in pregnancy) to their 'genetic' centile over the first few months of life. This may involve 'catch up' or 'catch down' growth.

Failure to grow is usually manifested in the first year of life as failure to gain weight appropriately (or 'failure to thrive'). The trigger for referral is usually 'crossing two major centile lines' (e.g. 75th through 50th to 25th). However, many such babies will simply be displaying 'catch down' growth. Actual loss of weight is always abnormal although transient loss may be explained by an acute illness and usually does not require investigation.

When assessing poor growth it is important to start with a good feeding history. The GP needs to know how much the infant takes and how often. This becomes more difficult as the child gets older and starts to take solids.

▷ Neonates should take 150 ml/kg/day (approximately 100 kcal/kg/day or 5 oz/kg/day) of milk.

▷ By 3 months the figure is probably about 100 ml/kg/day (3–4 oz/kg/day).

▷ Towards the end of the first year of life milk intake (including puddings and that poured onto cereals) should be about 0.5 litres (1 pint) per day.

▷ Solids can be measured in prepared jars (one per meal of the appropriate age preparation plus a pudding at one or two meals) or tablespoons (1–2 per meal at 6 months, 3–4 at 12 months).

Many feeding problems are behavioural (child or parents or an interaction of the two) but a history of vomiting and/or diarrhoea may imply food intolerance or a malabsorption syndrome. Coeliac disease can usually be excluded by a reliable blood test (99 per cent sensitivity for endomesial anti-bodies) although it is always confirmed by an intestinal biopsy. However, other intolerances (e.g. cow's milk protein intolerance – see Box 6.2) can only be excluded by an elimination diet that may have to be introduced for up to 6 weeks until symptoms fully resolve. Cystic fibrosis is normally detected on newborn screening while other malabsorption syndromes are very rare.

Always remember that some parents will deliberately harm, neglect or starve their children, leading to poor growth.

Box 6.2 ◡ *Cow's milk intolerance*

Intolerance to cow's milk protein (CMPI) affects 2–3 per cent of infants. This is of common concern to parents, and the following points are useful to bear in mind.

It may present with poor growth, poor feeding, vomiting, diarrhoea that may be bloody, and/or inconsolable crying.

CMPI is not the same as IgE-mediated cow's milk allergy, which typically presents with a rash and/or other more typical allergic-type symptoms. CMPI cannot be diagnosed with a skin prick or RAST test.

CMPI is also not the same as lactose intolerance, which is extremely rare in infants (although CMPI may cause a secondary lactose intolerance due to intestinal damage).

CMPI should be thought of as more like coeliac disease, although there is no blood test to confirm it and there is no evidence of extra intestinal manifestations.

If suspected the only diagnostic test for CMPI is to feed the child with a non-cow's milk-based formula and, if weaned, to avoid all foods containing milk, milk powder, whey protein, casein, etc. Non-cow's milk formulas available include hydrolysed formulas (e.g. Pepti, Nutramigen, Pregestimil) or, in severe cases, elemental formulas (e.g. Neocate).

Unfortunately these often taste unpleasant and parents report difficulty persuading infants to take their feeds (a significant problem in babies who are often already 'difficult feeders').

Beyond the age of 6 months soya-based formulas can be tried, although some children with CMPI will also have problems with soya protein.

Other mammalian milks generally confer no advantage over cow's milk, as is usually the case with lactose-free formulas, although occasional successes are reported.

CMPI will usually resolve as the child grows (20 per cent over the first year of life, 90 per cent by age 3 years) so parents should be encouraged to 'challenge' affected children with small amounts of cow's milk protein in the form of milk chocolate or biscuits containing milk every few months.

Chronic illness can also be a cause of poor growth. Tests for other systemic illness are usually carried out in secondary care but a systems-based history and examination may suggest a cause. Some examples are given in Table 6.5.

Table 6.5 ○ *Systemic approach to poor growth*

Cardiac	Classically a large ventriculoseptal defect will cause cardiac failure (tachypnoea, poor feeding, hepatomegaly) in the absence of a murmur
	Cyanotic congenital heart disease, especially tetralogy of Fallot and transposition with a large septal defect may go unrecognised for several months
	Children who have undergone surgery for complex congenital heart disease are frequently slow to grow
Respiratory	Chronic chest problems lead to increased metabolic rate and/or repeated vomiting
	Newborn screening may miss a child with cystic fibrosis, particularly one from a family that does not originate in Northern Europe
	(In older children aggressive treatment of asthma or any other condition with steroids may affect growth)
Renal disease	Chronic renal failure may occur secondary to renal dysplasia or severe vesicoureteric reflux
Endocrine	Hypothyroidism is the commonest endocrine cause of poor growth in older children but congenital hypothyroidism should be detected on newborn screening
	Growth hormone deficiency is sometimes recognised in the first year
Gastrointestinal	Liver disease and pancreatic insufficiency usually cause steatorrhoea
	Consider cow's milk protein and/or other dietary protein intolerance
	In a child who is weaned consider coeliac disease (especially if there is a family history)
	Remember pyloric stenosis can cause vomiting between birth and 3 months
Musculoskeletal	Neuromuscular weakness may lead to poor feeding, recurrent chest infections (some secondary to aspiration) and poor growth
Infection	Immune deficiency can lead to recurrent infections and poor growth. Consider HIV infection particularly in any infant from endemic areas
Social	Children from ethnic minorities with more pigmented skin are more prone to rickets
	Some cultures allow children to take a largely milk-based diet beyond the 6 months currently recommended in the UK. This can lead to severe iron deficiency

Acknowledgment

Thanks to Colette Colebourne, Newborn Hearing Screening Service, Local Co-ordinator, Burton-on-Trent.

Further reading

▷ Lingham S, Harvey D. *Manual of Child Development* Oxford: Churchill Livingstone, 1988.

References

1 • Griffiths R. *Griffiths Mental Development Scales* Henley: The Test Agency, 1996.

2 • Bellman M, Lingham S, Aukett A. *Schedule of Growing Skills II* London, UK: NFER-Nelson, 1996.

3 • Bayley N. *Bayley Scales of Infant Development* (second edn) San Antonio: The Psychological Corporation, 1993.

The ill child

Matthew Thompson and Anthony Harnden

7

Introduction

Children who present with acute illnesses are a very common part of general practice. As a GP trainee, one of the key skills that you have to develop is to be able to distinguish children with serious illnesses, who require urgent treatment and hospital referral, from the vast majority, who have less serious illnesses and who can be safely managed in the surgery. In addition there is also the large category of children about whom the parents are concerned but who are not ill.

The difficulty comes with developing the clinical skills that will let you differentiate children who require immediate treatment, and possibly hospital referral, from the majority who have minor or self-limiting illnesses.[1] Referring children unnecessarily is upsetting for parents and a poor use of hospital resources, while misdiagnosing rare conditions (such as meningococcal disease) is potentially devastating for the child, its family, and the GP.

This chapter uses some of the common childhood illnesses to develop a strategy for dealing with the ill child and covers some of the most important diagnoses to be familiar with.

Consider the following children who are typical of the ones seen in a routine GP surgery:

1 ▷ Hannah is 18 months' old and her mother called for an urgent appointment today. She had noticed that Hannah had been unwell for a day or so, with a fever, was off her food, and was less active than usual. She was very worried this morning when she noticed a rash on Hannah's body. She is worried that it could be meningitis.

2 ▷ You are working with your trainer in the out-of-hours surgery and the parents of Declan call. This is passed to you as an urgent call. This evening they had noticed that Declan, who is 18 months' old, suddenly developed a high fever. He was 'burning hot' and then seemed to have a 'twitch all over' for about 1 minute. He is breathing fine now and is wide awake. They are worried – should they call the ambulance? How can they prevent this happening again?

3 ▷ Jennifer is 3 years' old and has been complaining today of pain

when she passes urine. She is usually dry during the day but has been wetting herself today. She is slightly more irritable than usual today and off her food.

4 ▷ Jason aged 5 is brought in with a several-day history of runny nose, cough, slight fever, being off his food, and slight breathing difficulty. He has had several episodes of wheezing over his life. His parents thought that he was finding it difficult to get his breath last night.

5 ▷ Rachel is 7 years' old and has had several episodes of otitis media documented in her record. She comes in with her father saying that her left ear started really throbbing last night. She has had a slight cold for a few days, but no fever, and is feeling slightly better this morning after taking paracetamol.

Generally your approach to all acute illnesses in children will be similar:

▷ assess (fairly rapidly) how generally unwell they are
▷ determine what is the likely diagnosis and/or focus of their acute illness
▷ what treatment and advice is needed at this moment
▷ safety-netting so that if the child worsens or develops complications, the parents know what to look for and how to access care again.

The challenge with acutely unwell children is that you usually have limited opportunity to obtain additional investigations over and above your history and examination. Let us look at the general approach we recommend with children who are acutely unwell.

Box 7.1 ○ *General approach to children with acute febrile illness*

What key information should you get from the history?

Parents often focus on fever – perhaps because this is the most obvious physical sign of illness in many infections. Unfortunately, this is rarely useful enough on its own to discriminate how unwell a child is. Key things to ask about are the time course of the illness (a rapidly evolving infection in a systemically unwell child is of concern), as well as difficulty breathing, a rash, feeding problems, and risks for dehydration (vomiting as well as diarrhoea, no wet nappies). Try to gauge how active generally the child is. (Is the child playing just now? If not, what is the child doing?) Most parents do not bring their child to the GP each time they have an infection, so try to find out what is concerning them particularly this time.

What are the most important clinical features to look for?

You will gather the most useful information about the child from observing it in the initial few minutes of the consultation.[2,3]

continued

▷ Look for its overall activity: Does the child walk in or is it carried? Does the child start playing with toys? Is the child staring or not very alert? Or does it look at, smile or interact normally with its parent and/or you?

▷ Breathing – is the child breathing more rapidly than usual? Is it working hard to breathe, with intercostal and subcostal recession, grunting or nasal flaring?

▷ Colour – is the child very pale looking, or even ashen or cyanosed?

Which vital signs should you measure?

The National Institute for Health and Clinical Excellence (NICE) recommends measuring and recording heart rate, respiratory rate, temperature and capillary refill in every child who presents with acute febrile illness. In reality, most GPs do not carry these out on well-looking children, or may do them selectively on children who are looking generally unwell, or even to reassure the parents.[3,4]

▷ Fever can usually be detected by touching the child, but measuring temperature can be useful. You will need a fast-reading (i.e. 10 seconds) electronic axillary or tympanic thermometer.

▷ Respiratory rate is a useful sign of pneumonia and is best observed before you undress the child.

▷ Heart rate is difficult to measure accurately in children, due to fast rates and difficult-to-feel peripheral pulses. If you want to measure, then generally auscultation is the way. Tachycardia can merely be due to fever or anxiety, but can be an earlier sign of impending shock in children than blood pressure.

▷ Capillary refill time is not a very reliable physical sign of poor peripheral perfusion; however, it can be a concern if it is prolonged by more than 3 seconds. Cold extremities in a child with a fever can also indicate poor peripheral perfusion.

▷ Oxygen saturations – some GPs now use pulse oximeters, which provide heart rate in addition to oxygen saturations. Most children will have saturations over 94–95 per cent in primary care; if it is lower than this you must assess very carefully the overall respiratory status.

Let us consider each of the cases in turn.

Case 1: the possibility of meningitis in a child presenting with fever and rash

How common is this presentation?

Newly appearing rashes are very common in general practice. Most new rashes occur in children who are not unwell generally – such as *molluscum contagiosum* (umbilicated papules), impetigo (a small area of exudate with yellowish crusting on an inflamed base), or new onset (or exacerbation) of eczema.

Children who appear mildly systemically unwell with a rash could have one of the following:

▷ cellulitis, which is not usually associated with systemic illness, unless it is extensive, worsening or responding poorly to antibiotics

▷ chickenpox, which typically presents in children who are generally quite well, with only mild fever, and a blistering, itchy rash

▷ non-specific viral illnesses (such as enteroviral diarrhoea) that will have a blanching macular rash as part of their presentation

▷ hand, foot and mouth disease, caused by a coxsackie virus, which typically causes macules or blisters on the soles of the feet, palms and mouth

▷ scarletina – which is a typical fine papular rash (feeling like 'sandpaper') – occurs in children with current or recent streptococcal tonsillitis. It is usually treated with oral penicillin.

The causes of fever and rash that must not be missed

The challenge comes with children who present with a fever and rash, and who appear generally unwell. The differential diagnosis in these cases includes serious diseases such as meningococcal disease and Kawasaki disease, which we discuss below.

MENINGOCOCCAL DISEASE

The majority of cases of meningococcal disease occur in children under 5 years of age. A smaller peak occurs in teenagers of 15–19 years of age. Since the introduction of vaccination meningococcal serogroup C in 1999, 90 per cent of cases are now sporadic and caused by serogroup B. Meningococcal disease is the most common infectious cause of death in children in the UK. Almost one in ten children with meningococcal disease still die of this disease, and 8–15 per cent of survivors suffer from sequelae such as scars from skin lesions, amputations, or hearing loss. Yet it is rare, and most GPs will encounter this disease only once or twice in their careers. Nevertheless, it is vital to recognise this disease and refer children to hospital urgently as delays cause higher rates of complications and mortality.

DIAGNOSIS

The difficulty with diagnosing meningococcal disease in primary care is that many children do not exhibit the classic features of this disease in their early stages.[5] Some children will even present initially with upper respiratory tract or diarrhoeal symptoms – making it impossible to differentiate the disease from ordinary viral illnesses. The disease progresses rapidly from onset of first symptoms to hospital admission over 24 hours – therefore you should always take a history of rapid deterioration seriously, and offer a consultation to a child who appears to be deteriorating (even if the child was seen earlier in the day).

IMPORTANT CLINICAL FEATURES

Almost all children will have fever, while most will be drowsy, irritable and vomiting. Infants may be very sleepy, while older children and teenagers may appear confused (as if 'drugged'). Three early 'red flags' that may suggest meningococcal disease are leg pain, cold hands or feet, and skin pallor. One or more of these occur in three-quarters of children, at a median of 8 hours after the onset of illness. Children may have signs of meningism, but the 'classic' features of meningitis such as neck stiffness, photophobia and headache only occur in less than a third of children – so if they are not present you may not be reassured. You may find signs of reduced peripheral perfusion and impending shock, such as prolonged capillary refill time, tachycardia, or tachypnoea.

The most well-known sign of meningococcal disease, namely the typical haemorrhagic rash, can be petechial (non-blanching pinpoint red spots) or larger purpuric lesions. Although the rash usually appears in the first 12 hours, it may only be present in about half of children when they see their GP. Moreover, in the initial hours the rash may be blanching and macular in nature. Therefore it is worth undressing and examining the skin (including conjunctiva) to be sure this is not present.

TREATMENT

Your main priority with meningococcal disease is recognising it and referring children to hospital urgently. Current recommendations in the UK are to administer intramuscular benzylpenicillin to children in whom this disease is suspected.

Kawasaki disease and its diagnosis

Kawasaki disease is a rare but important disease in febrile children.[6] It is the commonest cause of acquired heart disease in children in the developed world. Treatment with immunoglobulins 7–10 days after the start of fever reduces the risk of the child developing coronary artery aneurysms. Children with Kawasaki disease are febrile and extremely irritable. You should suspect Kawasaki disease in a child who is irritable and has had a fever for at least 5 days. Other signs that may be present are: rash (described as measles-like, scarletiniform, or maculopapular), bilateral non-exudative conjunctivitis, changes to the lips or mouth (but not discrete ulcers), swollen, painful and reddened hands or feet (peeling may be a later sign) and cervical lymphadenopathy, which may be unilateral and large. Children may have incomplete Kawasaki disease so it is important to refer to a paediatrician for consideration of treatment even in the absence of a full house of clinical features.

Case 2: febrile convulsions in an 18-month-old

Incidence of febrile convulsions

Febrile seizures occur in 5 per cent of children under 5 years of age. The vast majority (nearly 90 per cent) last less than 10 minutes, but a third of children will have recurrent febrile seizures.[7]

What to do

Parents will be very worried and fearful after witnessing a scizure in their child. Children who have simple febrile seizures and who have a focus for their infection do not need further investigation. However, if the seizure has complex features (i.e. lasting longer than 10–15 minutes, multiple episodes within 24 hours, focal features), or if the child is unwell generally, then it should be referred acutely for paediatric assessment.

Assuming that these are not present, it is important to warn parents that febrile fits recur in one-third of children. Unfortunately there is no evidence that rigorous control of temperature will reduce the chance of recurrence.

Long-term risks

Parents may be worried about the long-term risks of epilepsy. There is a very marginal increased risk of epilepsy following simple febrile seizures. However, children who have had complex seizures do have a far higher risk of developing epilepsy.

'Fever phobia'

Fever is common. Parents are usually correct in knowing when their child has a fever. However, the actual level of fever recorded at home may be wildly inaccurate. Many of the inexpensive thermometers and devices (e.g. forehead strips) are not reliable. NICE recommends either an axillary electronic thermometer in children up to 4 weeks, and either an axillary thermometer (electronic or chemical dot single use) or infra-red tympanic thermometer in 4 weeks to 5 years. Above this age any method can be used, including oral.

Although serious infections are more common in children with higher temperatures, the majority of children with high fever will not have serious infections. Thus, you cannot use temperature alone as the discriminator between serious and mild infections. Many parents focus on the height of fever as the sole indicator of severity of illness. While accepting that fever is of concern to parents, you must make an overall assessment to determine the severity of illness.

Reducing temperature

There is some evidence that pyrexia is beneficial to fighting off infections, and that reducing fever can prolong infection. The presence of fever as such does not necessitate immediate reduction. However, children with fever are often uncomfortable and unhappy, and most parents want to do something to alleviate their distress.

Case 3: a 3-year-old girl with dysuria

Box 7.2 ○ *Recommendations to parents about reducing temperature*[8,9]
▷ Make sure that the child is not over-dressed (a common scenario). It is difficult for children who cannot remove clothing or bed clothes to regulate temperature.
▷ Suggest that the room heating is turned down or the windows are opened to reduce the room temperature.
▷ Tepid sponging is not recommended, as it is unpleasant to an already upset child and is not very effective. However, stripping off the child for a normal-temperature (i.e. not hot) bath can be a useful tip. This also allows the parent to see the child naked and observe any rashes.
continued

> ▷ Paracetamol or ibuprofen are available over the counter (or can be prescribed, though you will find parents prefer some brands as the flavours vary!). Ibuprofen has a longer duration of effect.
>
> ▷ If a child does not seem to respond to one antipyretic, then the other can be tried. NICE does not recommend using them alternately or at the same time. This is partly because there is no evidence that this is more effective, and also because parents may get confused about amounts they have administered.

Urinary tract infections (UTIs) are fairly common bacterial infections in children, which can range in severity from a mild, irritating cystitis, to a serious febrile illness due to pyelonephritis.

UTI presenting in children

In infants under 3 months, UTI is most likely to present as fever, vomiting, lethargy and irritability. It might also cause poor feeding and urine that smells offensive. In older infants and children, it may also cause fever, urine frequency and dysuria (in verbal children), but may also cause abdominal pain, vomiting, poor feeding, haematuria or smelly urine.

Diagnosis

Unlike UTIs in adults, it is important to try to confirm the diagnosis by getting a urine sample for dipstix, and to send for culture and sensitivity. Urine cultures are most important for:

▷ children under 3 years
▷ those with acute pyelonephritis
▷ where the risk of serious illness is high
▷ if a single dipstick test is positive for leucocytes or nitrites
▷ if clinical symptoms and urine tests do not seem to correlate
▷ if the infection does not respond to antibiotics within 1 or 2 days.

Children who are being potty trained can usually be persuaded to provide a sample – this is much easier at home into a recently sterilised and cleaned potty, or in the surgery in a cardboard vomit bowel. In children who are not toilet trained or infants, adhesive bags that fit over the genitalia are adequate; contamination can be reduced by having this put on after a quick bath, or after cleaning the perineum.

Treatment

Urgent referral is generally indicated for infants younger than 3 months with UTI, children with evidence of pyelonephritis or UTI who are systemically unwell (e.g. febrile, vomiting, irritable). All other children can be treated with 3 days of oral antibiotics; depending on your local microbiology recommendations this would usually be trimethoprim, nitrofurantoin, or amoxicillin-clavulanate. You should not delay treatment while waiting for the urine culture result, and should make sure that the parent will call (or the practice will call the parent) to let him or her know the result of the urine culture.

Follow-up

The recent NICE guideline on UTIs in children clarified the indications for imaging to detect underlying structural abnormalities of the renal tract:

▷ children with atypical UTI at any age (e.g. seriously unwell, abdominal masses, infection with non-*E. Coli* bacteria, failure to respond to treatment with suitable antibiotics) – ultrasound scan during the infection
▷ children younger than 6 months with first UTI responsive to treatment – ultrasound scan within 6 weeks of infection
▷ children younger than 3 years with atypical and/or recurrent UTI – DMSA scan 4 to 6 months after infection.

Case 4: a child with breathing difficulty

Assessment of severity of breathing in primary care

Problems with breathing are one of the most common reasons why parents present with a child for an acute illness. It is often quite difficult over the phone to fully assess the severity of respiratory distress, but always ask about rapid breathing, laboured breathing (which may mean something different to parents) and noisy breathing (including wheeze and stridor). Also it is useful to ask about feeding and hydration, and the child's overall level of activity.

Some of the clinical features that we look for at the start of the consultation are: a history of difficulty feeding due to dyspnoea; bouts of coughing or croupy cough (like a seal barking); or whether the breathing difficulty started acutely. (This might indicate possible choking or foreign body.)

Look at whether the child seems alert and responds to you. Is it drowsy and staring, or uninterested in surroundings? What is its colour like? Any cyanosis is immediately extremely concerning.

Assess the work of breathing before undressing the child (you might need to get the parent to loosen its vest or top to reveal some of the chest wall). The things to look for are breathing rate (count by observing not by auscultation), indrawing between the ribs (intercostal recession) or underneath the chest wall (subcostal retraction), supraclavicular recession, nasal flaring and grunting.

Only use your stethoscope when this is done. You should listen for crackles, bronchial breathing, wheezing noises, and symmetry between sides.

Signs of specific respiratory illnesses and what to do

PNEUMONIA [10]

▷ Consider this in a child who has fever, has tachypnoea and increased work of breathing (the absence of these almost excludes pneumonia).

▷ If there is severe respiratory distress or the child appears very tired then refer urgently.

▷ Mild pneumonia can be managed in the community. Use of oral amoxicillin is almost as effective as parenteral route.

BRONCHIOLITIS [11]

▷ Most cases occur between November and March in infants under 1 year of age.

▷ Presents with fever of a few days' duration, nasal discharge, and a wheezy cough. Wheezing may or may not be present. The features that distinguish bronchiolitis from bacterial pneumonia would be the absence of fever or signs of being systemically very unwell, and the presence of fine crackles all over the chest on auscultation.

▷ Only a few children with bronchiolitis will require admission – those who are dehydrated, or who are very tired due to significant tachypnoea or increased work of breathing, possibly requiring oxygen or ventilatory support, or those with apnoeic episodes, and any uncertainty of diagnosis.

▷ There is no specific treatment for bronchiolitis – maintaining feeds is vital in infants, while inhaled beta-2 agonists, steroids and antibiotics do not help. Some children will continue to have cough and wheeze for several weeks after bronchiolitis.[12]

CROUP [13]

▷ Usually occurs between 6 months and 3 years of age.
▷ The typical barking cough of croup usually occurs at night, and can be very alarming for children and their parents. Symptoms usually only last for 2 days.
▷ Severe respiratory distress, drooling, inspiratory stridor or dehydration indicate the need for urgent referral.
▷ A single oral dose of dexamethasone (0.6 mg/kg) improves symptoms and can reduce hospitalisation compared with placebo. A single dose of oral steroids is safe, and there are no other effective treatments in the community. Humidification (e.g. taking the child into the bathroom) is not really effective, and neither are oral decongestants, cough syrups nor antibiotics. Most chemists will be able to supply a single dose of dexamethasone – there is no need to prescribe a whole bottle as this is expensive. It is unclear whether prednisolone is as effective, which is a pity as it is much cheaper and more widely available.

Case 5: ear pain in an otherwise well child

Causes of ear pain

Acute otitis media (AOM) is common, and almost one in four children will have an episode before the age of 10 years. It peaks in children aged 3 to 6 and commonly starts with a history of URTI symptoms. AOM is painful. Older children may be brought in after crying with the pain, while preverbal children will often be fussy and miserable with a history of pulling, rubbing or holding that ear due to the pain. The ear drum may be cloudy, bulging or red. It can be extremely difficult to see the tympanic membrane in younger children, so the GP must make sure that the parent is holding the child firmly, and is using an otoscope with a bright enough light and correct size speculum. An ear discharge in this situation usually means that the ear drum has perforated, and this often coincides with the pain diminishing. It is always worth thinking about other causes of ear pain in children – these include otitis externa (usually more itchy than painful, often with a history of swimming, and not acutely unwell), referred pain from regional lymph nodes or dental problems, and temporomandibular joint pain (in teenagers).

Treatment of acute otitis media

Almost 80 per cent of children with AOM will be better within 3 days of seeing a GP. However, they may have had symptoms for several days prior to their consultation, with tired and fraught parents due to sleepless nights. It is important never to dismiss AOM in this situation – parents will not appreciate this! Although there is only a small amount of evidence that analgesics are important, either paracetamol or ibuprofen is worth using.

Rachel's mother states that she usually is given a script for antibiotics – will you do the same?

There has been a lot of research into the use of antibiotics for treating AOM. Overall, a Cochrane review found the number needed to treat (NNT) for one child to have reduced pain from AOM at days 2 to 7 was 15 (while the NNT for an adverse effect of antibiotics such as rash or diarrhoea was 17).[14] However, all children are not alike, and more detailed analysis of systematic reviews demonstrates a greater beneficial effect for children who are under 2 years of age, have bilateral AOM, or who have otorrhoea. For this group of children the NNT was only 4 for reduction of pain, fever or both at days 3 to 7.[15]

Clearly antibiotics have some effect, but the key issue is how great is the effect in a child, and what are the potential risks. We usually discuss antibiotics with the parents, and suggest whether their child is more or less likely to benefit from antibiotics based on the evidence. One option is to use a delayed script, with instructions to start this if the child is not improving. This can empower the parent, but also allows natural resolution of AOM and time for antipyretics. If you do use a delayed script, make sure you print it out on a separate prescription if you prescribe antipyretics at the same time.

Conclusions

This chapter has considered some of the common presentations of acute illness in children. Learning the skills to manage acute illness is often quite challenging for GP trainees, as the clinical scenarios are all very immediate, and there is always fear of missing serious disease.

Safety-netting is absolutely vital for children presenting with acute illnesses. Children who are obviously seriously unwell are not usually the ones who will challenge a GP. The difficulty comes with children who are somewhat unwell, or who have only one or two physical features of concern. In this situation providing safety-netting advice for parents – which includes specifically what clinical features to look out for, the time frame for these, and how exactly to access care – is fundamental.

Web resources and further reading

▷ Elliott EJ. Acute gastroenteritis in children (clinical review) *British Medical Journal* 2007; **334**: 35–40.

▷ National Collaborating Centre for Women's and Children's Health. *Clinical Guideline 47, Feverish Illness in Children: assessment and initial management in children younger than 5 years* London: RCOG Press, 2007. **www.nice.org.uk/Guidance/CG47** [accessed August 2009].

▷ National Collaborating Centre for Women's and Children's Health. *Clinical Guideline 54, Urinary Tract Infection: diagnosis, treatment and long-term management of urinary tract infection in children* London: RCOG Press, 2007, **www.nice.org.uk/Guidance/CG54** [accessed August 2009].

References

1 • Van den Bruel A, Bartholomeeusen S, Aertgeerts B, *et al.* Serious infections in children: an incidence study in family practice *BMC Family Practice* 2006; **7**: 23.

2 • Van den Bruel A, Aertgeerts B, Bruyninckx R, *et al.* Signs and symptoms for diagnosis of serious infections in children: a prospective study in primary care *British Journal of General Practice* 2007; **57**: 538–46.

3 • Thompson M, Mayon-White R, Harnden A, *et al.* Using vital signs to assess children with acute infections: a survey of current practice *British Journal of General Practice* 2008; **58**: 236–41.

4 • Harnden A. Recognising serious illness in children in primary care *British Medical Journal* 2007; **335**: 409–10.

5 • Thompson MJ, Ninis N, Perera R, *et al.* Clinical recognition of meningococcal disease in children and adolescents *Lancet* 2006; **367**: 397–403.

6 • Harnden A, Takahashi M, Burgner D. Kawasaki disease (clinical review) *British Medical Journal* 2009 (under review).

7 • Sadleir LG, Scheffer IE. Febrile seizures (clinical review) *British Medical Journal* 2007; **334**: 307–11.

8 • When the child has a fever *Drugs and Therapeutics Bulletin* 2008; **46**: 17–20.

9 • Hay AD, Costelloe C, Redmond NM, *et al.* Paracetamol plus ibuprofen for the treatment of fever in children (PITCH): randomised controlled trial *British Medical Journal* 2008; **337**: 1490–7.

10 • Margolis P, Gadomski A. The rational clinical examination: does this infant have pneumonia? *Journal of the American Medical Association* 1998; **279**: 308–13.

11 • Bush A, Thomson AH. Acute bronchiolitis (clinical review) *British Medical Journal* 2007; **335**: 1037–41.

12 • Townshend J, Hails S, McKean M. Diagnosis of asthma in children (clinical review) *British Medical Journal* 2007; **335**: 198–202.

13 • Cherry JD. Croup *New England Journal of Medicine* 2008; **358**: 384–91.

14 • Glasziou PP, Del Mar CB, Sanders SL, *et al*. Antibiotics for acute otitis media in children (Cochrane review). In: *Cochrane Database of Systematic Reviews*, issue 1: CD000219. Chichester: Wiley, 2004.

15 • Rovers MM, Glasziou P, Appelman CL, *et al*. Antibiotics for acute otitis media: a meta-analysis with individual patient data *Lancet* 2006; **368**: 1429–35.

Chronic disease in childhood

8

Tony Choules

Introduction

The GP can be confronted by children with chronic diseases at various stages of progression. In many cases it is the GP who will make the diagnosis and begin the long process of patient and parent or carer education. In some cases treatment will also be initiated but, increasingly, specific treatment of many chronic paediatric conditions is being co-ordinated by specialist teams. The GP must, of course, continue to provide support for the patient and family, adjusting treatment and managing crises often in liaison with a secondary care team. It is therefore important for the GP to understand the condition and its treatment, be able to recognise symptoms and adjust treatment or refer in a timely manner.

The chronic conditions covered in this chapter are: asthma, diabetes, arthritis, epilepsy and obesity. The principles generalise to other chronic conditions of childhood.

Asthma

Before reading on, take a minute to consider the case in Box 8.1

Box 8.1 ○ *Case history*

It is March and the worried parents of an 11-month-old boy bring him to see you. He developed a chesty cold at 5 months that took 3 weeks to settle. Since then he has had a cold every month. All the colds 'go to his chest', causing noisy breathing during the day and coughing at night. He has a cousin with asthma. The parents want something to be done.

What other information do you need to gather? Is this abnormal? What will you tell the parents? What treatment, if any, will you prescribe?

Asthma is a chronic inflammatory disorder that affects the airways. Inflamed airways are narrower and tend to react to certain stimuli by going into spasm. Symptoms produced include coughing (often a dry cough), wheezing, chest tightness and difficulty breathing.

The airway inflammation is reversible (in the early stages of the disease at least) with anti-inflammatory medications (steroids and leukotriene receptor antagonists [LRA]) and the spasm is reversible with bronchodilators (both short- and long-acting beta-2 agonists, and, sometimes, anticholinergic medication). Treatment is usually best given by the inhaled route, with the exception of montelukast and rescue steroids.

Diagnosis

Making the diagnosis in a teenager is usually easy. They present with typical symptoms (Box 8.2). Sometimes there is a clear history of trigger factors that exacerbate the symptoms. Wheeze may be heard in the acute phase.

Box 8.2 ○ **Symptoms of asthma**

▷ Wheeze.
▷ Shortness of breath.
▷ Chest tightness.
▷ Cough.

If there is doubt about the diagnosis then simple investigations can be used (Box 8.3).

Box 8.3 ○ **Investigation of asthma in the older child**

▷ >20 per cent variation in peak expiratory flow rate (PEFR) on at least 3 days per week over 2 weeks.
▷ >15 per cent increase in FEV_1 following beta-2 agonists or 2 weeks of oral steroids.

(The age at which spirometry becomes reliable varies between children – most 10-year-olds can do it and in specialist hands results can be obtained from children as young as 6 or 7.)

Diagnosis in a younger child (one who is too young for reliable spirometry) is usually more difficult and, as is often the case with children, may have to be made on 'the balance of probabilities'.

Although some children present with recurrent 'wheeze' it is helpful to be clear that the parents and the clinicians mean the same thing when they use this word. The term wheeze means a high-frequency 'whistle' and not just noisy, 'rattly' breathing.

Up to half of all children will wheeze at some time before they start school. Some of these children are thought to have small-calibre airways, making them prone to wheezing with minimal narrowing. Wheezing is usually associated with viral upper respiratory tract infections (URTIs) – so-called wheeze-associated viral episodes (WAVEs). Many children suffer from frequent URTIs, particularly those in daycare or with siblings in daycare/school (who can average 12 URTIs per year – one per month!) so recurrent wheezing (or at least chestiness) is fairly common.

Interval symptoms (those between URTIs) and symptoms that occur on exposure to cold, dust, etc. or on activity may sway one towards a diagnosis of asthma, as may a family or personal history of atopy (although, of course, not all asthma is atopic).

Persistent cough may be due to:

▷ gastro-oesophageal reflux
▷ rhinitis with postnasal drip
▷ foreign-body aspiration
▷ whooping cough (3 months' duration)
▷ congenital lung abnormality
▷ unresolved pneumonia.

111

It is important to distinguish these common symptoms from the less common *breathlessness*, which may be cardiac in origin (classically a large ventriculoseptal defect presenting at 2–3 months of age) or sadly, and increasingly, due to obesity (see below).

In many cases a trial of treatment is appropriate. If symptoms can be predicted then short-acting beta-2 agonists (salbutamol, terbutaline) can be tried. However, some infants do not respond to them or to inhaled anticholinergics (ipratropium bromide). Furthermore, symptoms are often frequent and unpredictable. It is therefore often appropriate to start inhaled steroids, preferably at the higher end of the starting-dose range suggested for the age of the child. Treatment can easily be stepped down if required. An alternative may be an LRA, e.g. montelukast. Failure of a trial of treatment should lead to a review of the diagnosis (Box 8.4, p. 112).

Initiating treatment

Treatment should follow the stepwise Scottish Intercollegiate Guidelines Network/British Thoracic Society (SIGN/BTS) guidelines (see Figure 8.1).[1] These differ a little for different ages. Treatment can be increased or reduced depending on control of symptoms. It is not necessary to start at Step 1 if clinical symptoms suggest a higher step is more appropriate.

Beclometasone or budesonide should start at 200–400 mcg for children under 12. Fluticasone and mometasone should be used at half the doses sug-

---

Box 8.4 ○ *Differential diagnosis of asthma*

Wheeze/noisy breathing
▷ WAVEs.
▷ Small airways.
▷ Recurrent respiratory tract illnesses.*

Shortness of breath/chest tightness
▷ Congenital cardiac/lung problem.
▷ Obesity.

Cough
▷ Foreign body.
▷ Whooping cough (3 months).
▷ Unresolved pneumonia.
▷ Gastro-oesophageal reflux.
▷ Postnasal drip.

---

* e.g. a child in daycare or with school-age siblings, cystic fibrosis, immune
deficiency or other lung disease.

---

gested for beclometasone or budesonide. Fluticasone is licensed from age 4
and mometasone from 12 years.

Steroids should generally be given by a pressurised metered dose inhaler
(pMDI) and large-volume spacer, which provide optimal lung deposition.
Older children with well-controlled asthma should be given a choice of
inhaler based on the premise that the most effective treatment is the one
the patient will take.

LRAs are an alternative at Step 2 or 3 in some cases. Long-acting beta-2
agonists (LABA) are not included in the SIGN guidance for those under the
age of 5 but can sometimes be helpful. The maximum recommended daily
dose of inhaled steroids is 800 mcg/day beclometasone for children 5–12 years
and 2000 mcg in older children/adults. Additional treatments to consider
if control is still poor are slow-release theophyllines, ipratropium bromide,
oral beta-2 agonists and in severe atopic asthma omalizumab.

For full details see: www.sign.ac.uk.

Ongoing care, counselling and crisis management

The aim of treatment is to eliminate all symptoms and the use of short-
acting bronchodilators, although some children will require them pre-
exercise or for URTIs.

You and the nursing team will come to know these patients well as you review them over the years. At review, all patients should be asked specifically about daytime symptoms, night-time symptoms and lifestyle compromise. It is recognised that patients with asthma develop tolerance to symptoms, treating them as normal. Specific questioning can help to uncover hidden symptoms. The Royal College of Physicians' (RCP) 3 Questions can help with this, as listed in Box 8.5.

Box 8.5 ○ **The RCP '3 Questions'**

▷ Have you had any difficulty sleeping because of your asthma symptoms?
▷ Have you had any of your usual asthma symptoms during the day?
▷ Has your asthma interfered with your usual activities?

Also consider more open questions such as 'If we could make one thing better for your asthma what would it be?'

Source: Measuring Clinical Outcome in Asthma: a patient focused approach London: Royal College of Physicians, 1999.

Where possible, spirometry provides an objective measure of control that is probably more reliable than a PEFR diary. Failure to respond to treatment as expected is usually due to poor concordance with treatment (including poor inhaler technique) but the possibility of incorrect or a concomitant diagnosis should be considered. Treatment can be stepped up and down as appropriate. At review a written plan should be agreed with the patient.

Inhaled steroids

Many parents express concerns regarding the use of inhaled steroids, especially when they may be used for several years. Some of these children may also be using steroid nasal sprays or eye drops as well as topical steroids, all adding to the total daily dose. How can a GP advise them?

With variable inhaler technique, different-potency steroids and different sizes of children establishing a 'safe' dose is difficult. Lipworth[2] provides the basis of the approach used in adults balancing dose response with potency. Priftis[3] suggests that a dose of 400 mcg/m^2 of betametasone (or equivalent) is probably a reasonable equivalent in children. This equates to a dose of 200 mcg for a pre-school child, 400 mcg for a school-aged child and 800 mcg for a teenager, and this is probably safe in most cases.

Although biochemical parameters may be measurable at lower doses, clinically measurable effects on growth (perhaps 1 cm/year) are probably more likely when these doses are exceeded. Catch-up growth should occur when the steroids are stopped, although uncontrolled asthma also affects growth.

Figure 8.1 ○ *Summary of stepwise management in children aged 5–12 years*

Source: Scottish Intercollegiate Guidelines Network/British Thoracic Society. *Guideline on the Management of Asthma.*[1] Used by permission of the BTS.

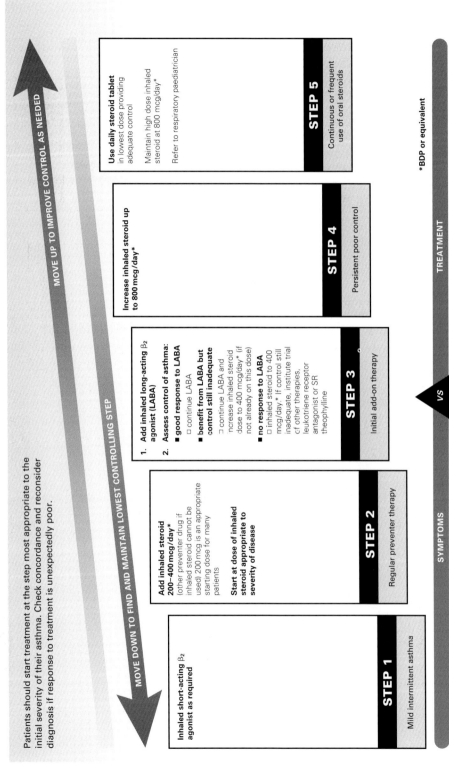

Patients should start treatment at the step most appropriate to the initial severity of their asthma. Check concordance and reconsider diagnosis if response to treatment is unexpectedly poor.

MOVE UP TO IMPROVE CONTROL AS NEEDED

MOVE DOWN TO FIND AND MAINTAIN LOWEST CONTROLLING STEP

STEP 1

Inhaled short-acting β₂ agonist as required

Mild intermittent asthma

STEP 2

Add inhaled steroid 200–400 mcg/day* (other preventer drug if inhaled steroid cannot be used) 200 mcg is an appropriate starting dose for many patients

Start at dose of inhaled steroid appropriate to severity of disease

Regular preventer therapy

STEP 3

1. Add inhaled long-acting β₂ agonist (LABA)
2. Assess control of asthma:
   - **good response to LABA**
     □ continue LABA
   - **benefit from LABA but control still inadequate**
     □ continue LABA and increase inhaled steroid dose to 400 mcg/day* (if not already on this dose)
   - **no response to LABA**
     □ inhaled steroid to 400 mcg/day.* If control still inadequate, institute trial cf other therapies, leukotriene receptor antagonist or SR theophylline

Initial add-on therapy

STEP 4

Increase inhaled steroid up to 800 mcg/day*

Persistent poor control

STEP 5

Use daily steroid tablet in lowest dose providing adequate control

Maintain high dose inhaled steroid at 800 mcg/day*

Refer to respiratory paediatrician

Continuous or frequent use of oral steroids

SYMPTOMS   vs   TREATMENT

*BDP or equivalent

Figure 8.2 ○ **Summary of stepwise management in children less than 5 years**

Source: Scottish Intercollegiate Guidelines Network/British Thoracic Society. *Guideline on the Management of Asthma.*[1] Used by permission of the BTS

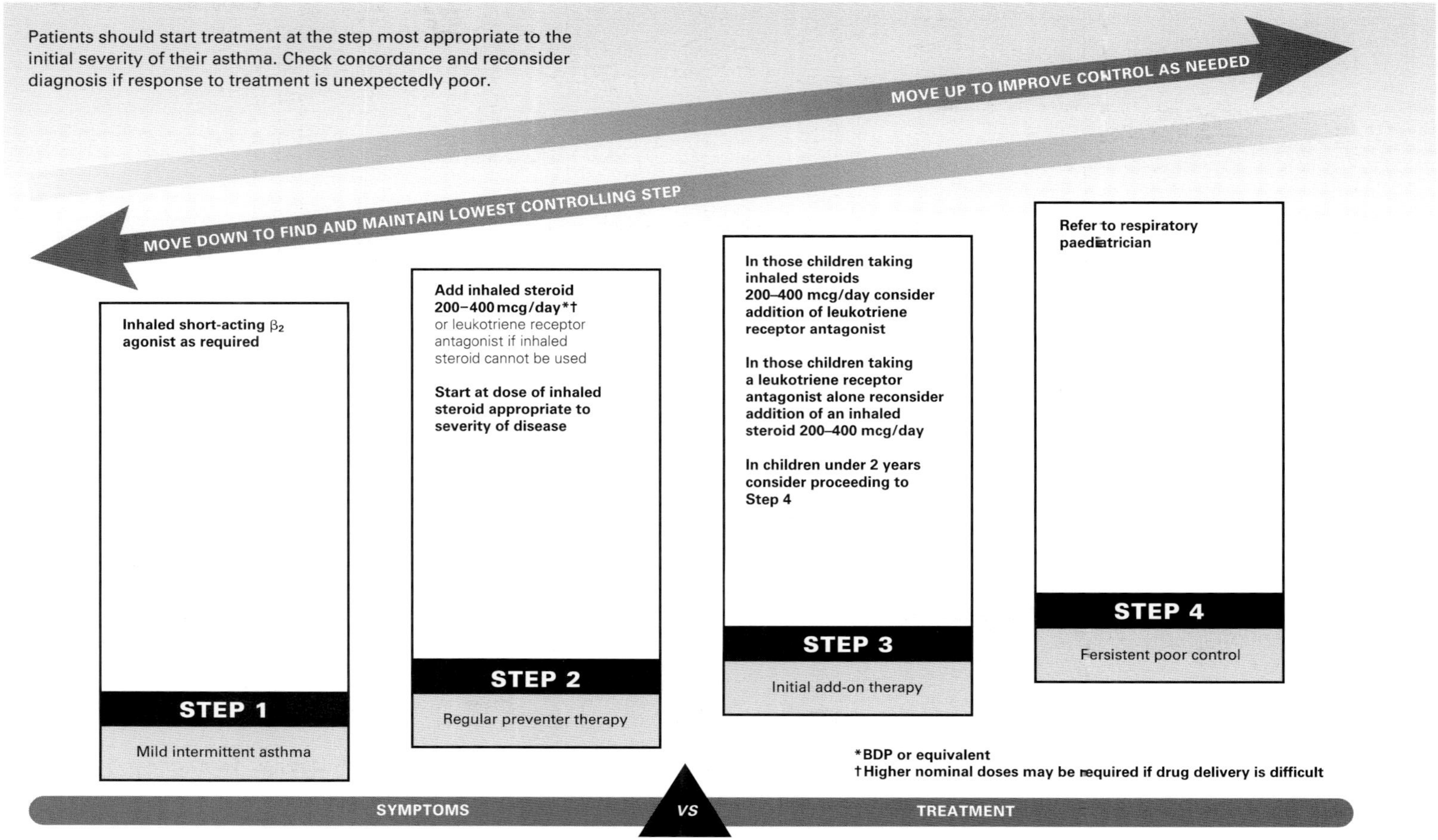

Patients should start treatment at the step most appropriate to the initial severity of their asthma. Check concordance and reconsider diagnosis if response to treatment is unexpectedly poor.

MOVE UP TO IMPROVE CONTROL AS NEEDED

MOVE DOWN TO FIND AND MAINTAIN LOWEST CONTROLLING STEP

STEP 1

Mild intermittent asthma

Inhaled short-acting β₂ agonist as required

STEP 2

Regular preventer therapy

Add inhaled steroid 200–400 mcg/day*†
or leukotriene receptor antagonist if inhaled steroid cannot be used

Start at dose of inhaled steroid appropriate to severity of disease

STEP 3

Initial add-on therapy

In those children taking inhaled steroids 200–400 mcg/day consider addition of leukotriene receptor antagonist

In those children taking a leukotriene receptor antagonist alone reconsider addition of an inhaled steroid 200–400 mcg/day

In children under 2 years consider proceeding to Step 4

STEP 4

Persistent poor control

Refer to respiratory paediatrician

SYMPTOMS   vs   TREATMENT

*BDP or equivalent
†Higher nominal doses may be required if drug delivery is difficult

115

Adrenal suppression leading to susceptibility to infection and 'Addisonian collapse' is usually associated with doses in excess of those in the guidelines, but can occur rarely on standard doses in children who presumably have increased sensitivity.

Fortunately, the suggested doses represent the flattening point of the dose–response curve. The higher doses at the higher steps in the guidelines may produce benefits in some children along with an increase in the risk of side effects. Increasing beyond the standard dose should be considered when control is poor, but failure to improve should trigger a return to the previous dose.

The small risk of side effects from steroids should be balanced against the risk of a severe (perhaps fatal) asthma attack, the psychosocial morbidity of uncontrolled asthma and potential long-term effects of airway remodelling. This includes failure to reach full adult lung function and probably increased respiratory morbidity in middle age and beyond.

116

Diabetes

Consider the case of Mary, described in Box 8.6.

Box 8.6 ○ *Case history*

Mary, aged 12, is brought to see you by her parents. She was diagnosed with Type 1 diabetes at the age of 6 years. Until 6 months ago she had good control. However, since then she has had problems with glycaemic control. She has 'gone hypo' twice at school, although generally her blood glucose levels are high.

How will you approach this problem? What are the possible causes?

Diagnosis

Most diabetes in childhood is Type 1, but the incidence of Type 2 diabetes in childhood is increasing as the epidemic of childhood obesity spreads.

The diagnosis of diabetes is usually relatively easy from a history of polyuria (sometimes manifest as bedwetting) and polydipsia (sometimes leading to odd behaviours) supported by a blood glucose level. At diagnosis there is usually a degree of dehydration, ketosis and metabolic acidosis. Even a well child should be referred urgently.

Treatment

Treatment is usually instituted in secondary care by a specialist paediatrician and diabetic nurse. Depending on the local set-up this might be as an in-patient or, sometimes, out-patient, but all children with suspected diabetes should be referred to secondary care because a significant amount of educa-tion is carried out by the specialist team in the first few days after diagnosis. Similarly, follow-up is usually secondary care-based with regular monitoring audited against national standards. Insulin is usually given in the form of a basal bolus regimen: a basal dose of a long-acting insulin (e.g. glargine) given once per day topped up at meal times with a bolus of rapid-acting insulin (e.g. lispro), the dose of this being adjusted according to the meal to be consumed. Standard mixes (e.g. mixtard) are also still used in some patients. However, the principle of dose adjustment remains the same with the longer-acting insulin being used to control preprandial glucose levels and the shorter-acting one to control postprandial levels. There is an increasing move towards using insulin pumps for more intensive management in some patients.

Ongoing care, counselling and crisis management

What about Mary? As with any chronic illness poor control is usually related to poor concordance with treatment. She is approaching the age where she might be starting to resent the perceived restrictions her illness causes and might be being teased by friends at school. The parents of her friends might be anxious about having Mary to stay the night on sleepovers, and this might be affecting her socially.

It is important to exclude physical causes for the poor control. A full examination to consider intercurrent illness will be important, as will be a review of height and weight and growth patterns.

The presence of lipodystrophy (hard lumps at overused injection sites) is one important physical sign. Rotation of injection sites to prevent this and allow more predictable absorption of insulin may resolve this problem.

Poor compliance with management and the accompanying lifestyle impli-cations are a common problem in teenagers with a chronic illness. Increas-ingly a psychologist forms part of the clinical team supporting children and families. Patients and parents may also manipulate treatment for secondary gain (both attention seeking and financial). In some cases obsessive control can lead to hypoglycaemia, particularly overnight. This may go unrecog-nised as the response by counter-hormones may produce rebound hyper-glycaemia on waking. Fear of hypoglycaemia, particularly at night, can lead to under-dosing. Reduction of insulin dosages to manipulate body image/weight is becoming an increasing problem.

Fear of hypoglycaemia is also a problem during an intercurrent illnesses, particularly when the patient is eating less. In this situation prevention of ketosis is important. Patients and parents should be encouraged to give insulin as usual during any illness (supported by high-calorie foods/drinks if required). Doses may need to be changed slightly up or down depending on glucose meter results.

Complications other than lipodystrophy and hypo/hyperglycaemia are rare in childhood, although screening is commenced at an early age. As with any chronic illness, as the child matures, he or she should become increasingly involved in discussion of the illness to provide education about disease control and the prevention of complications.

Arthritis

Box 8.7 contains another case to consider, before we go on.

Box 8.7 ○ *Case history*

Robin is a 6-year-old boy brought to you because he complains of being unable to walk. He was fine when he went to bed but when he tried to get up his leg hurt.

How will you approach this problem? What are the possible causes?

Arthritis is joint pain associated with objective signs (usually those of inflammation – dolour, rubor, calor, tumour (pain, redness, warmth, swelling) – and loss of function). Arthralgia is subjective joint pain.

Diagnosis

Joint pain and swelling are the usual presenting features of arthritis in childhood, although in one of the most commonly affected joints, the hip, swelling is not usually apparent. Combined with the inability of most young children to localise pain, this can lead to difficulties in diagnosis. In a young child loss of function (e.g. refusal to stand and/or walk) can be the only apparent sign. Classically, inflammatory arthritis causes more symptoms after a period of inactivity, e.g. morning stiffness.

As well as inflammatory arthritis, other conditions can present with pain localising in or near the joint (Table 8.1).

Table 8.1 ○ *Differential diagnosis of joint pain*

Diagnosis	Features	Additional aid to diagnosis
Septic arthritis	Usually unwell, febrile child and severe pain, can occasionally be multifocal	If uncertain then imaging and even exploratory surgery may be required
Trauma	Usually a history but beware non-accidental injury	History of previous trauma? Match between parents' story and findings?
Malignant bone pain	May waken child from sleep. Usually non-specific and generalised with marrow involvement; focal tumours are unusual and bony metastases very rare	A full blood count is usually carried out in children with bone/joint pain
Osteomyelitis/other bony lesions (e.g. osteochondroses such as Perthes)	History may be vague and unclear. Maintain a high index of suspicion if child persistently complains of inability to weight bear, especially for example at birthday parties	Early cases may be missed on X-ray, may require a repeat X-ray after 2 weeks (six if Perthes suspected) or require a bone scan to demonstrate
Congenital: joint laxity, undiagnosed dislocatable hips	Joint laxity can lead to joint pain that is usually worse on or after exertion. Undiagnosed developmental dysplasia of the hip (DDH) may lead to delayed walking	

Loss of function can also be due to other causes (Box 8.8).

Box 8.8 ○ *Differential diagnosis of loss of function*

▷ Neurological, e.g. Guillain-Barré, transverse myelitis, spinal lesion, postviral neuropathy.
▷ Muscular, e.g. Duchenne, viral myositis.
▷ Behavioural.

Inflammatory arthritis

There are two types of inflammatory arthritis that are important in childhood.

REACTIVE/POSTVIRAL/TRANSIENT SYNOVITIS

This is the commonest form of arthritis in childhood. Usually only one joint is affected and this is often the hip ('irritable hip'). The condition is self-limiting and parents may need a lot of reassurance that no further referral is needed. Treatment with non-steroidal anti-inflammatory medicine (e.g. ibuprofen) may be helpful if it is not contraindicated. Activity should be limited only by the child's symptoms.

A similar self-limiting arthritis may also be associated with Henoch–Schönlein purpura. In this case multiple joints can be affected and the characteristic rash will aid diagnosis.

JUVENILE IDIOPATHIC ARTHRITIS

This is currently the term used to encompass all forms of inflammatory arthritis in childhood. Previously the term Still's disease was also used. A number of phenotypes are recognised. The main diagnostic criterion is signs of joint inflammation for a period of longer than 3 months. Juvenile idiopathic arthritis, like many chronic inflammatory diseases, tends to have a course that waxes and wanes, although some patients are troubled by persistent symptoms. Treatment is instituted in a stepwise fashion beginning with non-steroidal anti-inflammatory medicine (increased to rheumatological doses if required, e.g. 60 mg/kg/day ibuprofen). Immuno-modulating drugs including steroids and methotrexate can be added if required. Local joint injection is being increasingly used. This should be supervised in secondary care. Other complications can arise, most notably inflammation in the eye leading to visual loss. Thus any patient with suspected juvenile idiopathic arthritis should also be referred to an ophthalmologist for regular screening.

In addition in primary care we may see other systemic diseases such as Crohn's, psoriasis or cystic fibrosis, which may cause an associated arthritis.

Ongoing care, counselling and crisis management

Ensuring appropriate doses of non-steroidal anti-inflammatory drugs is important. Analgesia may need to be escalated to opiates in certain crises, although this should only be done if a firm diagnosis has been made or pending the results of investigations. Steroids should only usually be instituted after specialist discussion. Physiotherapy, occupational therapy and orthotic support can be invaluable, and where a specialist service exists this is often provided as part of it. Liaison with schools can also be important, especially if mobility is impaired.

Epilepsy

An epileptic seizure occurs as a result of primary epileptic activity in the brain (hypersynchronous discharge of neurons). Seizures may be manifest as a constellation of activity that is classified as:

▷ motor (tonic-clonic, myoclonic, atonic)
▷ absence
▷ autonomic
▷ sensory.

Sometimes seizures that look exactly like epileptic seizures can be produced by other processes (e.g. febrile convulsions, hypoxic seizures following syncope) but these seizures are not epileptic. Epilepsy is defined as a condition in which the patient experiences recurrent epileptic seizures.

Consider the case outlined in Box 8.9 and reflect on what might be done next.

Box 8.9 ○ *Case history*

Henry, a 14-year-old boy, is brought to see you by his parents. He was recently at a show and was watching some video games on a big screen towards the end of the day. He suddenly slumped to the floor, jerked three times and wet himself. His uncle has epilepsy and parents fear their son is also suffering from the same condition.

Do you need any further information? What are the possible causes? Does he need any referral or investigation?

Diagnosis

The current National Institute for Health and Clinical Excellence (NICE) guideline suggests epilepsy in childhood be managed by a specialist.[4] Currently this is regarded as a paediatrician with an interest in epilepsy or a paediatric neurologist. The guidelines also suggest that a patient with suspected epilepsy should be seen in a 'timely manner' (usually taken to mean within a fortnight and certainly within 1 month).

The task of the GP is thus to recognise an epileptic seizure from other forms of 'funny turn' and make the appropriate referral. The diagnosis of epilepsy is made largely on the history given by the patient and observers (and, increasingly, via videos of the episode).

The specialist, as well as confirming the diagnosis of epilepsy, will attempt to define the epileptic syndrome affecting the patient to help direct treatment and give a prognosis (Box 8.10).

> **Box 8.10** ○ *Epilepsy syndromes and their differential diagnoses*
>
> ### Idiopathic generalised epilepsy
>
> This presents with generalised tonic-clonic seizures (GTCS – previously called 'grand mal') and sometimes with absences. GTCS may be confused with syncope or other cardiac event. Consider an ECG in all cases. Ten per cent of children who faint are incontinent and 50 per cent will have jerking of the limbs, though seizures secondary to syncope are usually very brief (<30 seconds). Children who faint usually feel an episode coming on (though this may be confused with an aura), look pale and have a fairly rapid (few minutes) recovery period.
>
> ### Typical childhood absences
>
> Previously called 'petit mal', these usually last no more than a few seconds. They can be associated with lip smacking, eye rolling and blinking. They can often be precipitated in the clinic by hyperventilation for 1–2 minutes. Typically children between the ages of 4 and 9 years are affected with the episodes eventually stopping, although some children will go on to develop other forms of epilepsy. Differential diagnoses include daydreaming, self-gratification, tics and hearing problems.
>
> ### Focal epilepsy
>
> This manifests in different ways depending on the part of the brain involved. Frontal-lobe seizures may affect behaviour, temporal and parietal lobe foci may cause strange behaviours (previously called 'complex partial'), those arising in the motor cortex may produce focal tonic and/or tonic-clonic movements, and sensory foci may give rise to sensory epilepsy. Clearly behavioural problems and tics are differential diagnoses; migraine should also be considered.
>
> ### Juvenile myoclonic epilepsy
>
> This usually presents in older children with focal seizures, typically on waking. Affected children may have jerky myoclonic movements in the morning leading to accusations of clumsiness. The condition is usually lifelong.
>
> ### Benign epilepsy with centro-temporal spikes
>
> Previously called benign rolandic epilepsy, this manifests as nocturnal seizures that may have an autonomic component. Daytime seizures may sometimes occur. Like most nocturnal epilepsy it is benign in that it is a transient condition and one that may not need treatment.

Ongoing care, counselling and crisis management

The long-term relationship a GP often has with a family will be vital in these cases, as several sessions might be needed to inform and educate the patient and his or her family regarding the diagnosis and treatment of the epilepsy. There still seems to be much stigma and fear attached to epilepsy, and education of others involved in the care of the child is often important. This may include relatives, friends, babysitters and teachers.

Discussion of the management of a seizure is also important, including keeping the child safe and protecting his or her dignity. Where appropriate (usually generalised tonic-clonic seizures) buccal midazolam may be prescribed to terminate a prolonged seizure, i.e. one lasting longer than 5 minutes. (This has largely replaced rectal diazepam.)

The child and carers should be aware of situations that are likely to trigger a seizure, such as tiredness, stress, alcohol consumption, missed doses of medication and intercurrent illness. Exposure to any of these or the particular trigger for an individual child should be minimised where possible, whilst trying not to limit the child's lifestyle too much. Unless the epilepsy is photosensitive (which is rare) there is no need to avoid strobe lighting and night-clubs.

Persistence of seizures despite medication should lead to a review of medication, with probable increase in the dose up to the recommended maximum or the emergence of side effects. There is little place for the measurement of anticonvulsant level other than to check concordance with medication.

Children and carers should be made aware that significant physical harm from epilepsy is rarely due to the seizure itself, and the risks of bathing, swimming alone, climbing without safety equipment, riding a bike and, in some cases, crossing the road should be discussed. With good seizure control (usually defined as seizure freedom for 6 months) some of these cautions may be relaxed.

Some parents fear the risk of a fatal seizure and will have read about Sudden Unexpected Death in Epilepsy (SUDEP). Barring accidents, death due to a seizure is extremely rare in otherwise healthy children with well-controlled epilepsy. Those in whom the epilepsy is well-controlled for a period of 2 years may choose to reduce and stop treatment if the natural history of their epilepsy is one of complete remission.

Obesity

This is perhaps the most difficult condition of all to manage. Consider Jake, in Box 8.11.

Box 8.11 ○ *Case history*

Jake is a 15-year-old boy who is brought to see you because he is breathless when he runs around. There is a strong family history of asthma and you ask him to complete a peak flow diary. When he returns 2 weeks later the diary shows no evidence of asthma. His height is 160 cm and his weight is 80 kg.

How will you approach the issue of his weight? What will you do about it?

Diagnosis

The NICE guideline suggests that obesity requires intervention when a child's body mass index (BMI) is above the 91st centile.[5] (BMI is calculated as weight in kg divided by height in cm².)

Assessment of co-morbidities is recommended where the BMI is above the 98th centile. See Box 8.12.

Box 8.12 ○ *Co-morbidities of obesity*

▷ Hypertension.

▷ Dyslipidaemia.

▷ Hyperinsulinaemia.

▷ Type 2 diabetes.

▷ Psychosocial problems (low self-esteem, bullying).

▷ Exacerbation of underlying respiratory illness (e.g. in asthma).

Ongoing care, counselling and crisis management

In most cases obesity is simply caused by consuming more calories than are expended. The aim of management is to reverse this cause or, at least, prevent further weight gain.

Rarely there is an underlying endocrine cause (e.g. hypothyroidism, Cushing's), although this is often suspected by parents or the patient themselves.

Assessment should include review of diet and lifestyle. In some cases simple dietary interventions are possible, such as changing to diet drinks, using semi-skimmed milk and swapping sugary breakfast cereals for low-sugar ones. However, dietary measures alone are not usually sufficient and lifestyle changes will need to be suggested and negotiated with the child and family.

The current guidelines for exercise in childhood suggest 60 minutes of exercise per day (and also add that some children will need more than this!). There is an emphasis on family involvement and a reduction in TV watching/computer games. Realistic goals should be set (often the maintenance of weight as the child grows) and praise given for success. Drug treatment is only recommended in children in extreme circumstances (e.g. sleep apnoea, orthopaedic problems).

Looking after children who have chronic conditions

Although the management of children with different chronic conditions requires different treatments there are some fundamental issues affecting the management of all conditions.

Primary care management

The degree to which chronic childhood conditions are managed within primary care varies depending upon the condition. Asthma management is covered in detail in this chapter as many GPs manage childhood asthma to differing levels. Referral is suggested at around Step 3 of the SIGN/BTS guidelines, although some practitioners refer earlier than this and some later. Referral should be guided by personal experience. Obesity is managed largely in primary care, although increasingly obesity clinics are being developed. Most of the other conditions are managed largely in secondary care, particularly when a specialist nurse is available for patients and parents to contact. In these cases GPs should be aware of possible complications and when to reassure and when to seek support. National guidelines for most chronic conditions recommend that practices keep a register of patients with the condition to ensure regular review and allow audit.

As years go by, children and young adults with chronic conditions are bound to have other problems that GPs are called upon to help with, such as infective illnesses, musculoskeletal injuries, behavioural problems and contraceptive advice. The continuity of care afforded by registered lists allows GPs to develop good relationships with young patients that can be built on in these circumstances.

Person-centred care

Carers require clear explanations and, in many cases, written guidance. Contact a Family (www.cafamily.org.uk) may be a useful resource to put families in contact with others in a similar situation. As children become older they need to understand their condition with a view to taking on responsibility for self-management. They should be allowed to assert their independence and be supported in adjusting their treatment where possible to suit their lifestyle. Becoming independent and conforming to peer pressure can be major challenges. Overall, adolescence can be viewed as a series of hurdles that can become more difficult for a young person who also has to deal with a chronic illness. Variations in treatment regimens, for example by the use of long-acting/slow-release medications, may be helpful.

The GP may also be able to help by providing information or facilitating access to it, perhaps via the internet. DIPEx (www.dipex.org.uk) provides patient perspectives on illness that may be helpful.

Helping to support young people may involve helping them to discuss their condition with friends who may be the first on-scene when a crisis occurs. A knowledge of the effect of the conditions on potential career choices and disability legislation may also be useful.

Specific problem-solving skills

Although the GP may not manage all of the chronic conditions of childhood alone, he or she is usually the first point of contact with healthcare services when a chronic condition is developing. It is thus important for the GP to recognise the symptoms of chronic conditions, differentiating where possible the chesty child from the asthmatic, picking out the baby with Kussmaul breathing in the bronchiolitis epidemic, separating the child trying to avoid games lessons from the child with juvenile idiopathic arthritis, reassuring the fainting teenager who has jerked twice during an episode that he or she does not have epilepsy, and introducing the concept of nutrition and exercise to the obese family.

A comprehensive approach

Children with chronic illnesses also need the usual services provided to other children, including vaccination, health promotion and contraceptive advice. This must be given in the context of the illness and its treatment (e.g. most antiepileptics reduce the effectiveness of the oral contraceptive pill). Support with non-healthcare issues such as schooling, transport, mobility seating, etc. may also be required.

The GP may also be asked to contribute to the Educational Statementing process (www.direct.gov.uk/en/Parents/Schoolslearninganddevelopment/SpecialEducationalNeeds/index.htm) and/or attend multidisciplinary meetings to discuss the child's needs with other professionals including psychologists, physiotherapists, occupational therapists, etc.

Community orientation

The GP is often best placed to manage the child and family overall. Being aware of the social context in which the family lives can provide an insight into likely concordance with medication, including family issues affecting control of the child's illness. Sadly some parents manipulate illness in small children for financial gain. Similarly children may manipulate their own illness for social gain. The GP may be best placed to make appropriate referrals for secondary care for both the chronic condition and its psychosocial effects.

A holistic approach

The GP can support the child and family through investigation, diagnosis and treatment to promote physical, mental and emotional wellbeing. They must also support transition to adult care when required.

Case study

Katie is 16 years' old and comes to see you with her mother. She was diagnosed with epilepsy at 10 years of age and has been taking carbamazepine 400 mg b.d. since then. She tells you that her last seizure was over 2 years ago. As her epilepsy was well controlled she has not attended her out-patient appointments with the paediatrician. A letter in the notes states that she has been discharged from hospital care for three failed appointments.

Katie is keen to stop her medication. What do you do?

Stopping medication after 2 years' seizure freedom is reasonable in many cases. However, some types of epilepsy are unlikely to remit. You need to know the type of epilepsy she has to provide advice and allow her to make a more informed choice. Depending on the type of epilepsy it might be reasonable to reduce her medication over the next 2 to 3 months. Seeking specialist advice from a paediatrician with an interest in epilepsy or, at this age, a neurologist is probably sensible.

You discuss Katie's request with the on-call paediatrician who agrees that it is reasonable to stop her medication.

What do you need to tell Katie and her family?

After warning of the risks of further seizures and possible difficulty regaining control you agree that she should tail off her carbamazepine over 3 months. You warn of the precautions to take like not bathing alone, not climbing too high and the effects that having a seizure will have on obtaining her provisional driver's licence. You tell her that if after 2 years she has not had a fit it is reasonable to assume that she has probably grown out of her epilepsy.

Four months after the initial meeting she returns with a story of seizures in the morning that leave her unsteady on her feet and clumsy for an hour or two and then tired through the day. As a result she is keen to restart medication.

What would you do?

Restarting the antiepileptic medication is probably reasonable although, depending on the type of epilepsy, carbamazepine may not be the best choice. However, as it has worked well before and the family are very keen, you suggest she restart her carbamazepine 400 mg b.d.

Three days later she is brought to see you by her mother. She feels very unwell. The unsteadiness is worse, now lasting all day, and has reached the point where she has difficulty standing up. She is also complaining that she is seeing double.

What has happened?

Katie has carbamazepine toxicity. Her previously induced hepatic metabolism has returned to a normal state since stopping the carbamazepine and the previous dose she needed to remain stable now represents an overdose. You tell her to stop the carbamazepine and agree to send her for urgent secondary care opinion.

Do you refer her to her old paediatric consultant or to an adult neurologist?

The decision largely depends on patient choice, although it may be influenced to some extent by local services. If she is likely to have ongoing problems then adult services may be more appropriate.

Katie is seen by the specialist who makes a diagnosis of juvenile myoclonic epilepsy and transfers her to sodium valproate. Unfortunately a month later she has a generalised tonic-clonic seizure lasting 7 minutes while shopping with her sister. She was taken to the emergency department by ambulance but recovered spontaneously. The emergency department team suggested she contact you over the next few days and she comes in with her mother the next day.

What do you advise?

Buccal midazolam can be used to terminate prolonged seizures. You prescribe some and show her mother how to use it. You also increase her sodium valproate.

A month later she comes to see you again. She has been avoiding school in case she has another seizure.

Can you help?

A number of problems arise around school. Sometimes there is anxiety from the school about taking a child with seizures. Many teenagers are anxious about the possibility of having a seizure in front of their friends. In these cases the school nurse (or epilepsy nurse, if there is one) can be very helpful. She may be able to help Katie speak to her friends and, if necessary, teach them how to administer the buccal midazolam. Most peer groups among teenagers are very accepting.

Further advice can be obtained from: www.epilepsy.org.uk.

Web resources and further reading

▷ Appleton R, Gibbs J. *Epilepsy in Childhood and Adolescence* [third edn] London: Martin Dunitz, 2003.

▷ Arthritis Research Campaign, **www.arc.org.uk** [information on arthritis including a rapid clinical assessment tool for joint problems in children (pGALS)] [accessed August 2009].

▷ British Paediatric Neurology Association, **www.bpna.org.uk** [runs Paediatric Epilepsy Training (PET) courses] [accessed August 2009].

▷ British Thoracic Society. *British Guideline on the Management of Asthma: a national clinical guideline* Edinburgh: SIGN, 2008, **www.brit-thoracic. org.uk/ClinicalInformation/Asthma/AsthmaGuidelines/ tabid/83/Default.aspx** [accessed August 2009].

▷ Cochrane Collaboration, **www.cochrane.org** [accessed August 2009].

▷ e-Learning for Healthcare, **www.e-lfh.org.uk** [has an online package covering adolescent health] [accessed August 2009].

▷ Epilepsy Action, **www.epilepsy.org.uk** [advice for patients and carers about epilepsy] [accessed August 2009].

▷ International League Against Epilepsy, **www.ilae.org** [provides the definitive resource for specialists including definitions and descriptions of seizure types/syndromes] [accessed August 2009].

▷ McCann L, Wedderburn L, Hasson N. Juvenile idiopathic arthritis *Archives of Disease in Childhood: education and practice edition* 2006; **91**: 29–36.

▷ National Institute for Health and Clinical Excellence. *Obesity: the prevention, identification, assessment and management of overweight and obesity in adults and children* London: NICE, **www.nice.org.uk/ guidance/CG43** [accessed August 2009].

▷ Rudolf M. The obese child *Archives of Disease in Childhood: education and practice edition* 2004; **89**: 57–62.

▷ Scottish Intercollegiate Guidelines Network. *British Guideline on the Management of Asthma: a national clinical guideline* Edinburgh: SIGN, 2008, **www.sign.ac.uk/guidelines/fulltext/101/index.html** [accessed August 2009].

▷ Stokes T, Shaw E J, Juarez-Garcia A, *et al. Clinical Guidelines and Evidence Review for the Epilepsies: diagnosis and management in adults and children in primary and secondary care* London: RCGP, 2004, **www.nice.org.uk/ guidance/CG20** [accessed August 2009].

▷ Syncope Trust And Reflex anoxic Seizures, **www.stars.org.uk** [information on neurocardiogenic syncope, reflex anoxic seizures, etc.] [accessed August 2009].

Acknowledgements

I would like to thank Jane Humphries, Paediatric Diabetes Nurse, and Gill Reed, Paediatric Respiratory Nurse, both of Queen's Hospital, Burton upon Trent.

References

1 • Scottish Intercollegiate Guidelines Network, British Thoracic Society. *British Guideline on the Management of Asthma: a national clinical guideline* [revised edn] Edinburgh: SIGN, 2009, www.brit-thoracic.org.uk/ClinicalInformation/Asthma/AsthmaGuidelines/tabid/83/Default.aspx [accessed August 2009].

2 • Lipworth B J. Airway and systemic effects of inhaled corticosteroids in asthma: dose response relationship *Pulmonary Pharmacology* 1996; **9**: 19–27.

3 • Priftis K, Milner A D, Conway E, *et al.* Adrenal function in asthma *Archives of Disease in Childhood* 1990; **65**: 838–40.

4 • Stokes T, Shaw E J, Juarez-Garcia A, *et al. Clinical Guidelines and Evidence Review for the Epilepsies: diagnosis and management in adults and children in primary and secondary care* London: RCGP, 2004, www.nice.org.uk/guidance/CG20 [accessed August 2009].

5 • National Institute for Health and Clinical Excellence. *Obesity: the prevention, identification, assessment and management of overweight and obesity in adults and children* London: NICE, www.nice.org.uk/guidance/CG43 [accessed August 2009].

Psychological problems

9

Kay Mohanna

According to Hall and Elliman, emotional and behavioural disorders in children and young adults are common, but service provision is often inadequate and fragmented.[1] Some of the conditions considered in this chapter are not behavioural problems in the true sense of being psychological issues. However, they are certainly behaviours that cause families to have problems.

Consider the following cases that might occur in any routine GP surgery.

1 ▷ Mrs MacDonald has booked an appointment to see you on her own to discuss Ryan, her 7-year-old son. Ryan has a Cub Scout adventure weekend booked in 2 months' time. The problem is he is still wetting the bed nearly every night. Mr and Mrs MacDonald have got in the habit of 'lifting' Ryan and carrying him to the toilet about 11 p.m. every night to try and ensure he has a dry night, but they are worried that this will not be possible when he is away from home without them. They are worried that Ryan will be embarrassed, or that they will have to cancel the trip.

2 ▷ Sam is 6 years' old and is described as a bright and happy child. For the past 3 months he has been soiling his pants and from time to time has taken to hiding dirty underwear under his bed. He plays happily with the toys in your surgery and does not seem anywhere near as bothered about this as his mother, who is very anxious for a referral to a paediatric gastroenterologist. She is convinced that something serious is the matter with his bowels.

3 ▷ Wayne is a patient you have known for some time who had a very troubled childhood. He comes to see you in an outrage that his 7-year-old son, Kyle, has been 'accused' of being a bully. Kyle has been excluded from school. Wayne feels that Kyle is a very sporty child, keen on boxing, which he and Kyle do together at a local club, and that his high-spirited encouragement of the other boys on the football team has been misinterpreted.

4 ▷ Lottie is 11. She has always done well at school and enjoyed life in her small primary school in the village. Her mother Kate comes to see you at the end of her tether because it is becoming increasingly difficult to get Lottie to go to school now she has moved to secondary

school. Every morning there are tears and difficult scenes when Lottie clings to her mother at the school gate. It is nearly the end of term and recently Kate has stopped trying to take Lottie. The headmistress has now written to the family about Lottie's non-attendance.

It would be an unusual surgery if all these came in on the same day and, if they did, a general practice specialty registrar would be forgiven for emerging at morning coffee somewhat dazed and drained! However, these are all very familiar scenarios – not rare encounters in general practice.

Increasingly, GP trainees enter medical school as graduates, are older and with some life experience under their belt. They may well have a family of their own and have encountered some of these issues first hand. This is important, because the first step will be to reassure parents that they are not alone, that there are interventions that can be tried and that the GP understands the impact such disruptions can have on family life.

In addition GPs may be more familiar with folk remedies and 'parent-lore' than their counterparts two decades ago might have been when medical students usually went straight to medical school and entered several years of training before starting families. They often felt very ill-equipped to deal with some of these areas.

We will consider each of the cases in turn, consider how best to get to grips with all the issues they present, list which red flags might need to be carefully excluded and importantly consider which members of the primary healthcare or multidisciplinary team might need to be involved.

Ryan MacDonald – a case of primary nocturnal enuresis

What is the size of the problem?

Bedwetting is more common in boys than girls. Most girls are dry at night by age 6 and most boys are dry by age 7. Boys make up 60 per cent of bedwetters overall and make up more than 90 per cent of those who wet nightly. Often there is a family history and sometimes asking if the father was also 'late' becoming dry at night can help demonstrate to the child he or she is not that unusual and that it will get better, just like Dad.

Approximate bedwetting rates are:

▷ age 5 ▶ 20 per cent
▷ age 6 ▶ 10–15 per cent
▷ age 7 ▶ 7 per cent

▷ age 10 ▶ 5 per cent
▷ age 15 ▶ 1–2 per cent
▷ age 18–64 ▶ 0.5–1 per cent.[2]

So again, it might reassure Ryan to know that in his class of 30 children at least one other boy probably has a similar problem. The GP could tell Ryan that, just as he does not know which classmate that is, the others do not know about him either. So long as he has a shower every morning when he has a wet night, the issues of smelling of urine and subsequent teasing at school will not arise.

Under the age of 6 or 7, no treatment is indicated. Indeed, most children will grow out of it. Children 5 to 9 years' old have a spontaneous cure rate of 14 per cent per year. Adolescents 10 to 18 years' old have a spontaneous cure rate of 16 per cent per year. So the chances for Ryan achieving a run of dry nights on his own are high.

But Mrs MacDonald is fed up with all the laundry, is worried that there is something wrong with Ryan and there is the Cub camp to worry about as well.

Ryan has primary nocturnal enuresis. The commonest cause at this age is developmental delay – he has just not yet reached the age when he has acquired full bladder control. He is on the cusp of the age when it is appropriate to do more than await spontaneous resolution, however, especially with the impending trip.

So what are you going to do to help?

▷ Talk to Ryan. Place him at the centre of the consultation and try to find out his level of understanding and what bothers him most. Talk to the parents, understand Ryan's birth order and experiences of any siblings. Does he have a younger sister who is already dry?
▷ Examine Ryan for growth and weight, and his abdomen to rule out a palpable bladder or constipation. It would be very unlikely that a mild form of spina bifida had been missed earlier in life, but this could cause lack of bladder control.
▷ If Ryan looks fit and well, and is doing well at school, it is unlikely that there are any serious physical problems. Bedwetting is a very uncommon presentation of diabetes mellitus at this age but dipstick urinalysis is important to exclude an infection or glycosuria. Also check the specific gravity of an early-morning specimen. Diabetes insipidus and failure of enhanced antidiuretic hormone (ADH) production should be excluded. Check for albumin too. Chronic renal failure, though again rare, can present with failure of concentration of urine and bedwetting.

133

▷ Clarify what the family have tried or are currently doing. Fluid restriction is not recommended, nor is lifting (taking the child from its bed and sitting it on the toilet whilst drowsy or still asleep), which simply teaches children that they need not attend themselves to the signals from a full bladder. However, Ryan should make sure his bladder is empty before going to bed, not drink to excess after 6 p.m. and avoid fizzy drinks and others that contain caffeine.

The most appropriate form of treatment in the longer term is behavioural modification. And in this consultation you will be keen to develop a rapport with Ryan, gain his trust and use that as the basis for the next stage.

However, first, there is Cub camp to worry about and a quick fix is needed. Desmopressin is a synthetic analogue of ADH and has become the most popular form of drug treatment for this condition. The oral route should be used for this indication (not nasal). It is important to avoid fluid overload after taking it – so in this case fluid restriction is appropriate and intake should be limited to 250 ml.[3]

Tricyclic antidepressants, usually in the form of amitriptyline or imipramine, may be used for their anticholinergic side effects. They can cause behavioural disturbance. Relapse often occurs on stopping them and they should not be used for longer than 3 months without reassessment.

Either of these should work, and there is time to try out treatment before the important trip. Success will bolster Ryan's self-esteem and you will go up in the estimation of both mum and Ryan for solving the problems.

However, success will be short-lived unless you follow it up. Drug treatments cannot be continued for longer than 3 months. You therefore need to develop your second line of attack.

Behavioural modification is by two main forms. Star charts reward success and build the child's self-esteem. Ask Ryan to bring his in and praise any dry nights. Ignore the wet ones. Enuresis alarms work by waking the child as soon as the alarm senses wetness, so that he will stop urinating, go the toilet and learn to recognise the nocturnal sensation of a full bladder.

A Cochrane review found poor evidence to support hypnosis, psychotherapy, acupuncture and chiropractic.[4]

Sam – a boy with encopresis

What is the size of the problem?

Encopresis, or faecal soiling, is estimated to affect 1 to 2 per cent of children under 10. Ninety per cent of cases of soiling or 'accidents', such as children having their bowels open behind the sofa, are due to constipation with overflow diarrhoea.

It is another condition that is more common in boys – perhaps between 2 to 6 times more common than in girls in the same age group.

There are some conditions, Hirschsprung's disease and spina bifida for example, that can cause constipation or encopresis, but these are rare. Similarly it is on rare occasions associated with child sex abuse.

The GP should start as always by taking a good history. Any number of things including diet, illness, decreased fluid intake, or limited access to a toilet (or avoiding the toilets at school) can set the cycle up. Once a child starts to hold onto stools, increased fluid is removed in the colon and large, dry stools accumulate. These may be difficult to pass, leading to anal fissures, and the subsequent pain of opening the bowels perpetuates the avoidance and the problem. The bowel distends and the normal sensation of the call to stool is impaired.

Some children may develop chronic constipation after stressful life events such as a divorce or the death of a close relative, or when a new baby joins the family. Although encopresis is not thought to be part of the oppositional–defiance spectrum it might be a symptom of depression or anxiety. This underlying issue might also need to be addressed for successful treatment.

Sam's mother may well have looked this condition up on the web. She is very concerned and is keen to be referred to a paediatrician. It is however a condition that responds well to simple treatment and can be managed in primary care if you can establish trust and a good relationship.

Treatment involves emptying the overloaded colon with laxatives or enemas, regular use of stool softeners and a training programme. This encourages the child to sit on the toilet and try to empty the bowels, perhaps after breakfast to capture the benefit of the gastro-colic reflex, in a regular pattern.

Kyle – the class bully

Despite Wayne's views, his son has been found by his teachers to be a bully. Teachers are rightly increasingly intolerant of aggressive 'teasing' when it extends to a distressing level and much more likely these days to intervene and act when children are suffering at the hands of a bullying classmate. It is worth considering what effect Kyle's home circumstances are having on him developing as a bully as often the behaviour is a perpetuation of how the bully is him or herself being treated.

Might some of your patients be Kyle's 'victims'? What is the size of the problem?

In their series *Mental Health and Growing Up,*[5] the Royal College of Psychiatrists quotes recent surveys in the UK that show that one in four primary school pupils and one in ten secondary school pupils are being bullied.

The Royal College of Psychiatrists offers advice to parents and this is reproduced in Box 9.1 to help you work out how to support children who report they are being bullied.[5]

Box 9.1 ○ *Advice to parents*

Be open to the possibility that your child might be being bullied. Some parents may not think of bullying as a possible reason for their child's distress.

Listen. One of the most important things you can do is to listen to your child if they say they are being bullied. It can be very difficult for them to talk to anyone about it.

Take your child seriously. Many children suffer in silence for a long time before they tell anyone.

They may be ashamed, embarrassed, and may believe that they deserve it. Many children are frightened of telling because they fear the bullies will find out and hurt them even more. It can take great courage to tell an adult.

Do not blame the child. Being bullied is not their fault (although they may think it is).

Reassure them that they were right to tell you.

Do not promise to keep the bullying a secret, something must be done about it. Reassure your child that you, and the teachers, will make sure that things do not get worse because they have told you. Tell the school so they can stop it. Teachers don't always know that a child is being bullied. Find out if there is an anti-bullying programme in the school.

Talk with your child and work out ways of solving the problem.

Include your child in decisions about how to tackle the problem. For example, work out some practical ways for them to stop the bullying. You might discuss what they should say back if they are called names, or where it's safe to go at playtime.

Source: Royal College of Psychiatrists.[5]

As the GP, remember that there are other agencies you can call on for help. School nurses often offer counselling sessions, especially in secondary schools. In severe cases an educational psychologist will be able to offer help and advice.

As for Kyle? He is at risk of entering the spiral of aggression and violence that perhaps he too has experienced at home. You will need all your listening skills and open communication style to work out whether he is at risk. If you have any concerns, consider taking advice under the child protection procedure (see Chapter 4).

Lottie – a child refusing to go to school

For many children who are refusing to go to school, it may be that it is a natural extension of the bullying discussed above. In Lottie's case it appears to have started just after the move to secondary school and such transition phases are commonly affected. It is not uncommon for children to take a while to adjust to the larger scale of the new environment. In this case, things have escalated and Lottie finds herself coming to the attention of the authorities through non-attendance.

What is the size of the problem?

School refusal affects 3–5 per cent of all school-aged children. The most common ages for school refusal are between 5 and 6, and between 10 and 11. Children who suffer from school refusal tend to be average or above average in intelligence.

This is different from truancy, which is more common in adolescents who are rebelling against authority or unhappiness and is sometimes associated with antisocial or illegal activity. These young people act deceitfully to avoid going to school and instead spend time with their friends. Lottie is quite open and her behaviour might have several causes:

1 ▷ Separation anxiety
2 ▷ Being a high achiever at primary school, she may fear being a small fish in a big pond
3 ▷ Fear of bullies or a certain teacher
4 ▷ Concerns about making new friends or leaving old friends behind.

It might also arise out of such issues as changing for PE lessons, using showers after games or the additional pressure of more formal examination systems.

Lottie may have symptoms that are similar to those of anxiety. She may complain of nausea, tummy ache, headache, fatigue, dizziness or vague and non-specific aches and pains. If she can be persuaded to go into school these often settle rapidly. Similarly if she is allowed to stay at home, they will settle, only to recur the next morning. Sometimes if anxiety is episodic or situational, she may have symptoms that recur at certain times in the day and this may be sufficient for teachers to send her home.

There are several symptoms associated with school refusal that point to a more general anxiety syndrome. Try to get to the bottom of this with questions to Lottie's mother, such as the following.[6]

▷ Does she feel unsafe staying in a room by herself?

▷ Does she display 'clinging' behaviour?

▷ Does she voice worries and fears about her parents dying or about harm to herself?

▷ Does she shadow you around the house?

▷ Does she have difficulty going to sleep, or have nightmares?

▷ Are there exaggerated, unrealistic fears of animals, monsters, burglars, or of being alone in the dark?

Management can be challenging. Often by the time the parents bring their child to see you behaviours have become entrenched and tempers are frayed. The following advice to parents might help.

1 ▷ They must continue to try to take their child to school. Home schooling is rarely the answer as this can perpetuate maladaptive responses to stressful situations.

2 ▷ It is important to inform the child calmly that they will definitely be back to collect the child after school, and then leave quickly.

3 ▷ If complaints of illness are the excuse for not attending school, parents should use common sense about whether the child is ill, get them checked by the GP if they are not sure, and then take them back into school the same day if the child is well.

4 ▷ Try talking to determine the underlying reason for refusal. This involves being open, and building a safe, caring environment, rather than an angry or punitive one. This is not always easy when parents are rushing to get to work themselves, so needs to be done outside of school.

5 ▷ Talk to the child's teacher about developing an appropriate plan to solve any issues that come from such discussions.

If the refusal to attend school is becoming a habit, or if the child is very distressed every morning, you may need to consider referral for cognitive behavioural therapy. This is likely to include relaxation therapy, advice about better coping skills, working on improving social skills and building different strategies to minimise or manage stress.

Conclusion

This chapter has considered some of the common childhood behavioural problems in general practice. The GP is a central figure in co-ordinating services for such children, and close working with health visitors and school nurses is important. At all times building good relationships with parents is essential.

Specialist, expert help is available from paediatricians, educational psychologists, social workers and child and adolescent psychologists. The GP needs to know when and for which children and young people it is appropriate to refer.

There are many other conditions not covered in this chapter and further guidance can be found on such issues as temper tantrums and breath holding, as well as mental illness, from the Royal College of Psychiatrists (see further reading below).

Conditions that present less commonly and are likely to need psychiatric intervention are covered in Chapter 10.

Web resources

▷ Royal College of Psychiatrists. *Mental Health and Growing Up* series of factsheets, **www.rcpsych.ac.uk/mentalhealthinformation/ mentalhealthandgrowingup.aspx**:

1 ☐ The restless and excitable young child
2 ☐ Good parenting
3 ☐ Dealing with tantrums
4 ☐ Behavioural problems and conduct disorder
5 ☐ ADHD and hyperkinetic disorder
6 ☐ Stimulant medication for hyperkinetic disorder and attention deficit hyperactivity disorder
7 ☐ Sleep problems in childhood and adolescence
8 ☐ Children who soil or wet themselves
9 ☐ Children who do not go to school
10 ☐ The child with general learning disability
11 ☐ Specific learning difficulties
12 ☐ Understanding autism and Asperger's syndrome
13 ☐ Worries and anxieties – helping children to cope
14 ☐ Divorce or separation of parents – the impact on children and adolescents
15 ☐ Death in the family – helping children to cope
16 ☐ Parental mental illness – the problems for children
17 ☐ Domestic violence – its effects on children
18 ☐ The emotional cost of bullying
19 ☐ Child abuse and neglect – the emotional effects
20 ☐ Traumatic stress in children – how parents can help

21 ☐ Schizophrenia

22 ☐ Bipolar affective disorder (manic depression)

23 ☐ Obsessive-compulsive disorder in children and young people

24 ☐ Eating disorders in young people

25 ☐ Suicide and attempted suicide

26 ☐ Deliberate self-harm in young people

27 ☐ Chronic physical illnesses: the effects on mental health

28 ☐ Medically unexplained physical symptoms

29 ☐ Chronic fatigue syndrome (CFS): helping your child to get better

30a ☐ Alcohol and drugs: what parents need to know

30b ☐ Information about drugs: what parents need to know

31 ☐ Child and adolescent psychiatrists: how they can help

32 ☐ Coping with stress

33 ☐ Psychotic illness

34 ☐ Depression in children and young people

35 ☐ Worries about weight

36 ☐ Drugs and alcohol

References

1 • Hall D, Elliman D. *Health for All Children* (4th edn) Oxford: Oxford University Press, 2003.

2 • www.pediatriceducation.org/2005/04/04 [accessed August 2009].

3 • Glazener C M, Evans J H. Desmopressin for nocturnal enuresis in children (abstract). In: *Cochrane Database of Systematic Reviews*, issue 3: CD002112. Chichester: Wiley, 2002.

4 • Glazener C M, Evans J H, Cheuk D K. Complementary and miscellaneous interventions for nocturnal enuresis in children (abstract). In: *Cochrane Database of Systematic Reviews*, issue 2: CD005230. Chichester: Wiley, 2005.

5 • Royal College of Psychiatrists. Factsheet 18: the emotional cost of bullying: for parents and teachers. In: *Mental Health and Growing Up* (3rd edn) London: RCPsych. 2004, www.rcpsych.ac.uk/mentalhealthinfoforall/mentalhealthandgrowingup/18bullyingandemotion.aspx [accessed August 2009].

6 • American Academy of Child and Adolescent Psychiatry. www.aacap.org/cs/root/facts_for_families/children_who_wont_go_to_school_separation_anxiety [accessed August 2009].

Mental health problems

10

Kay Mohanna

Major psychiatric illness in children is uncommon. However, there are some conditions that present not infrequently and in this chapter we will consider some of the conditions that are most likely to present in general practice.

Autistic spectrum disorder

The NHS Direct Health Encyclopaedia defines autistic spectrum disorder (ASD) for parents as 'A lifelong condition that affects how a person communicates with, and relates to, other people. It also affects how they make sense of the world around them.'[1]

The spectrum, also known as pervasive developmental disorders (PDDs), includes Asperger's syndrome. These patients tend to have average, or above average, intelligence, but still have difficulty interacting with others and making sense of the world. On the whole, sufferers from autism also have a learning disability.

Estimates vary but between 1 and 3 per cent of the UK population are thought to suffer with ASD, with boys up to four times more likely to be affected than girls. Some of the high-performing Aspergers may be undiagnosed so prevalence may be much higher. There is a 2–8 per cent risk of a sibling also being affected.

The symptoms can be grouped into three areas: interaction with others, verbal and nonverbal communication and behaviour. Parents may become aware that their child, although initially making good developmental progress, appears to be lagging behind his or her peers, until the discrepancy becomes very clear and help is sought. Unusual, repetitive behaviours that can be difficult for parents to understand, and attempted modification of which can lead to aggressive outbursts, can be distressing.

Possible indicators of ASD are listed in Box 10.1 (p. 142).

Although a child with ASD may attend mainstream school, they may need extra support or specialised schools. They are likely to have a statement of special educational needs and may need speech and language therapy to enable them to understand the nuances of interaction and communicate with others (see Chapter 11).

Box 10.1 ○ *Possible indicators of ASD*

▷ Does not babble, point, or make meaningful gestures by 1 year of age.

▷ Does not speak one word by 16 months.

▷ Does not combine two words by 2 years.

▷ Does not respond to name.

▷ Loses language or social skills previously acquired.

▷ Poor eye contact.

▷ Does not seem to know how to play with toys.

▷ Excessively lines up toys or other objects.

▷ Is attached to one particular toy or object.

▷ Does not smile.

▷ At times seems to be hearing impaired.

Problems that may accompany ASD

Sensory problems

Children with ASD seem to lack the normal checks and balances that allow them to integrate information from their senses. They may be extremely sensitive to loud noises or bright lights or light touch, yet tolerate extreme pain and discomfort. They may respond with symptoms of high anxiety or distress to sudden movements yet engage in repetitive self-harm behaviour such as head banging and be at risk of burns without feeling the pain.

Seizures

One in four children with ASD develops seizures, often starting either in early childhood or adolescence.

Fragile X syndrome

This disorder is the most common inherited form of mental retardation overall and affects about 2 to 5 per cent of people with ASD. It is important to have a child with ASD checked for fragile X in order to give accurate genetic counselling about future pregnancies. Being sex linked, there is a 50 per cent risk of recurrence of fragile X syndrome in a male sibling.

Tuberous sclerosis

Tuberous sclerosis is a rare genetic disorder but 1 to 4 per cent of people with ASD also have this.

Management

Certain aspects of the condition, such as seizures, obsessive behaviour, anxiety and restlessness, can be managed with medication. Early diagnosis is important because, although the management options are limited, tailored educational programmes have the best chance of allowing a child with ASD to integrate into society. Structured and individually planned programmes are important. Naturally, in a condition that can be devastating for families and for which there is no cure or specific treatment, all sorts of interventions are tried by parents, including self-help such as homeopathy and dietary manipulation.

143

It is worth adding a word about children with ASD who are approaching adolescence. This can be a difficult time, and behaviour may become increasingly disturbed as the young person begins to notice that he or she is different from those around him or her. The changeover from child to adult psychiatric services can mean a new set of professionals to get to know just at a time when stability and familiarity are important. Cognitive behavioural therapy (CBT) might help to ease the adjustment.

The role of the GP includes acting as a signpost to sources of support. One such is the National Autistic Society at www.autism.org.uk.

Attention deficit hyperactivity disorder

Attention deficit hyperactivity disorder (ADHD) and attention deficit disorder (ADD) refer to a range of problem behaviours associated with poor attention span. The prevalence is hard to be certain of but it is thought to affect 1–2 per cent of the population, and boys are more commonly affected than girls. Over 50 per cent of children will not persist with symptoms into adult life, but those that do may go on to exhibit depression or antisocial behaviour and poor impulse control.

The diagnosis can be difficult to make as these children may appear intelligent, active and interested in what is going on. The British Psychological Society criteria for diagnosis are listed in Box 10.2 (p. 144).[2]

Box 10.2 ○ *Diagnosis of ADHD*

Attention difficulties

A child must have exhibited at least six of the following symptoms for at least 6 months to an extent that is unusual for its age and level of intelligence.

▷ Fails to pay close attention to detail or makes careless errors during work or play.

▷ Fails to finish tasks or sustain attention in play activities.

▷ Seems not to listen to what is said to it.

▷ Fails to follow through instructions or to finish homework or chores (not because of confrontational behaviour or failure to understand instructions).

▷ Disorganised about tasks and activities.

▷ Avoids tasks like homework that require sustained mental effort.

▷ Loses things necessary for certain tasks or activities, such as pencils, books or toys.

▷ Easily distracted.

▷ Forgetful in the course of daily activities.

Hyperactivity

A child must have exhibited at least three of the following symptoms for at least 6 months to an extent that is unusual for its age and level of intelligence.

▷ Runs around or excessively climbs over things. (In adolescents or adults only feelings of restlessness may occur.)

▷ Unduly noisy in playing, or has difficulty in engaging in quiet leisure activities.

▷ Leaves seat in classroom or in other situations where remaining seated is expected.

▷ Fidgets with hands or feet, or squirms on seat.

Impulsivity

At least one of the following symptoms must have persisted at least for 6 months to an extent that is unusual for its age and level of intelligence.

▷ Blurts out answers before the questions have been completed.

▷ Fails to wait in lines or await turns in games or group situations.

▷ Interrupts or intrudes on others, e.g. butts into others' conversations or games.

▷ Talks excessively without appropriate response to social restraint.

Source: netdoctor.co.uk.[2]

Management

A child who has ADHD, and its family, will need the support of professionals and other parents. A child psychologist or educational psychologist should be involved from the beginning and a structured individualised programme of behaviour support will be needed. Occasionally medication can help. It is important to exclude other conditions that might be mistaken for ADHD such as tic disorders, Tourette Syndrome and certain forms of epilepsy first, but methylphenidate and atomoxetine might be helpful. Dexamphetamine is an alternative second-line treatment for those who do not respond. Tricyclic antidepressants, such as imipramine, have also been used with some success. All of these treatments need to be accompanied by a comprehensive treatment programme and so should be started by a specialist in ADHD. They are likely to be needed well into adolescence or even adulthood.

National Institute for Health and Clinical Excellence (NICE) guidance has been developed for the treatment and management of ADHD.[3]

Parental support can be gained from the charity ADHD Information Services at www.addiss.co.uk.

Depression, suicide and self-harm in childhood

Depression affects 2 in every 100 children under 12 years' old, and 5 in every 100 teenagers. Although, just as with adults, low mood can be intermittent and relate to situational disturbance, young people can become significantly depressed and mentally ill, and can resort to self-harming behaviour and can die at their own hands.

Depression can present as school refusal and social isolation, reduced involvement in previous hobbies and activities, insomnia, excess sleeping and eating disorders.

Deliberate self-harm can include: overdosing with prescription and non-prescription medication, alcohol or other chemicals such as household cleaners; hitting, cutting or burning the skin; pulling hair or picking skin; or self-strangulation. Children in abusive situations or who are isolated are more at risk and self-harm is commonly precipitated by arguments with others.

For those whose symptoms are severe and persistent, CBT for 3 months can help and antidepressant medication may also be needed. Antidepressant medication needs to be taken for 6 months after the young person feels better. Although SSRIs are not licensed for use in the under-18s, fluoxetine can be used, and others in this class if started and monitored in secondary care. Research has shown that the benefits outweigh the risks.

The risk of suicide is higher when a young person:[4]

▷ is depressed, or when he or she has a serious mental illness
▷ is using drugs or alcohol when he or she is upset
▷ has tried to kill him or herself a number of times or has planned for a while about how to die without being saved

▷ has a relative or friend who tried to kill themselves.

Self-harming behaviour and suicide attempts should never be dismissed as 'a cry for help' or 'attention seeking'. Sometimes they occur at times of increased distress, such as after an argument or bereavement when they can be considered impulsive. It might be tempting to think of these as one-off episodes, especially since the young person might feel embarrassed at the fuss he or she feels has been caused and deny suicidal intention. They are better characterised as 'attention needing'. These young people may have significant mental illness that they are unable to express or access help for in any other way. All such attempts require psychiatric evaluation.

Eating disorders

Anorexia nervosa and bulimia nervosa are more common in girls, but can occur in boys, when it is often overlooked. Men and boys account for an estimated 5 to 15 per cent of patients with anorexia or bulimia and an estimated 35 per cent of those with binge-eating disorder. Over time these conditions become less amenable to intervention and modification, and can become life threatening. They may coexist with other, treatable, conditions such as substance abuse, anxiety and depression.

The signs of anorexia or bulimia as listed by the Royal College of Psychiatrists are reproduced in Box 10.3.[5]

Box 10.3 ○ *Signs of eating disorders*
▷ Weight loss or unusual weight changes.
▷ In girls, periods becoming irregular or stopping.
▷ Missing meals, eating very little and avoiding 'fattening' foods.
▷ Avoiding eating in public; secret eating.
▷ Large amounts of food disappearing from the cupboards.
▷ Belief in being fat when underweight.
▷ Exercising excessively.
▷ Becoming preoccupied with food; cooking for other people.
▷ Going to the bathroom or toilet immediately after meals.
▷ Using laxatives and vomiting to control weight.

If untreated, there is a risk of infertility, osteoporosis, stunted growth and even death.

The reasons why these conditions start are poorly understood. They may begin as a concern for body image but in these patients this progresses to a form of body dysmorphism and a distortion of perception of body shape. There are likely to be both behavioural and psychological components to the condition. For most patients there will be physical and psychological components to the treatment regime.

Recognising eating disorders

Symptoms and signs of eating disorders are listed in Table 10.1

Table 10.1 ○ **Symptoms and signs of eating disorders**

Anorexia nervosa	Bulimia nervosa
Thinning of the bones (osteopenia or osteoporosis)	Chronically inflamed and sore throat
Brittle hair and nails	Swollen glands in the neck and below the jaw
Dry and yellowish skin	Worn tooth enamel and increasingly sensitive and decaying teeth as a result of exposure to stomach acids
Growth of fine hair over body (lanugo)	Gastro-oesophageal reflux disorder
Mild anaemia, muscle weakness and loss of muscle	Intestinal distress and irritation from laxative abuse
Severe constipation	Kidney problems from diuretic abuse
Low blood pressure, slowed breathing and pulse	Severe dehydration from purging of fluids
Drop in internal body temperature, causing a person to feel cold all the time	
Lethargy	

Patients are likely to need specialist support. This may mean from the child and adolescent psychiatric team, and the patient may be allocated a community psychiatric nurse for support and surveillance. Increasingly, specialist eating disorder units are being set up where the complex physical effects can be monitored and treated in addition to psychological treatment. Antidepressants are often used but cognitive behavioural work is important.

Help is available at the registered charity BEAT at www.b-eat.co.uk.

Obsessive–compulsive disorder

Obsessions (intrusive thoughts that might make a person feel silly) and compulsions (repeated or ritualistic activities) are common. If they start to affect how the person gets on with others, or interferes with life, it might mean the start of an obsessive–compulsive disorder. For these patients anxiety levels mount unless the ritualised activities are carried out. Parents trying to intervene and minimise these patterns may well be met with aggressive outbursts, tears of frustration and extreme agitation.

For all children at times of stress such as parental separation or starting school these might become more common, but this is usually short lived. Patterns of behaviour might include counting or organising possessions and toys. For some children it can progress and seriously affect day-to-day activities. Repeated hand washing or checking that lights have been turned off might start to interfere with getting to school on time.

Treatment regimes include CBT aimed at altering the way these children think about the outcomes of their actions. Medication in the form of fluvoxamine or sertraline under the supervision of a psychiatrist can result in an improvement for up to two-thirds of patients, but this is unlikely to be maintained if CBT is not used as well.

Psychotic illness

Schizophrenia is the most common form of psychosis and affects one person in every 100 people of all ages. The incidence of new cases is very low and very rare before puberty. It is most likely to start between the ages of 15 and 35 years, although it can occur in younger children. Bipolar affective disorder affects fewer than one in 100 people of all ages. It is extremely rare before puberty, but becomes more common during teenage years and adult life.

Schizophrenia is characterised by delusions, thought disorder and hallucinations, and also by negative symptoms. Young people with schizophrenia may express bizarre fears due to their delusions and can withdraw from friends and family, and spend a lot of time on their own. They may lose interest in hobbies, activities and studies. It is easy to see how a young person, finding it difficult to concentrate because of auditory hallucinations and unable to communicate effectively due to thought disorder, will become increasingly frightened and of extreme concern to his or her family.

Bipolar affective disorder is difficult to diagnose, especially because the most common age for a young person to become affected is in adolescence when mood swings are more common anyway. The following list might help make the diagnosis if certain characteristics are extreme or out of step with the young person's personality:

▷ depression, moodiness, irritability, excitement or elation
▷ very rapid speech and changes of subject
▷ loss of energy or excessive energy
▷ change in appetite and weight
▷ sleep disturbance
▷ neglect of personal care
▷ withdrawal from family and friends, or excessive sociability
▷ feelings of guilt, hopelessness, worthlessness, or inflated ideas about self or abilities
▷ reckless behaviour, spending excessive amounts of money, sexual promiscuity
▷ unusual or bizarre ideas, beliefs or experiences
▷ preoccupations with death, suicide attempts.

Parents may present to the GP on their own, unable to get the young person to acknowledge there is a problem. Information may need to be gathered from school or youth workers. You will want to know whether there is any history of drug use as psychotic illness can arise following experimentation with drugs. Such drug use may interfere with the prognosis.

YoungMinds Parents' Information Service provides information and advice on child mental health issues at www.youngminds.org.uk.

Changing Minds: a multimedia CD-ROM about mental health is a resource available from the Royal College of Psychiatrists and is intended for 13–17-year-olds (at www.rcpsych.ac.uk/campaigns/changingminds/materials/cdroms.aspx). It covers addiction, stress, eating disorders, depression, schizophrenia and self-harm.

Involving others

As with other psychological or mental health conditions in primary care, management plans for all these conditions must include appropriate input from a wide range of healthcare professionals. The role of the GP is to stay alert to the possibility that the symptoms being described by worried parents, or by young people themselves, might start off as part of a normal spectrum but may represent conditions needing significant help.

Referral to Child and Adolescent Mental Health Services (CAMHS) should be considered in the following circumstances:[6]

149

▷ where the young person is displaying signs of suicidal intent
▷ where specialist assessment of the young person is needed (e.g. psychotic symptoms, attention deficit/hyperactivity disorder [ADHD])
▷ where the young person is likely to require medication, and treatment will need to be initiated by a specialist (e.g. depressive disorder in a child, severe obsessive–compulsive disorder)
▷ where the young person is so disabled that he or she cannot go to school or see friends
▷ if the young person or parent requests a referral
▷ where primary care or other options have failed.

Referral to other agencies may also be necessary. For referral to social services the criteria include the following:

▷ any form of suspected abuse
▷ when a young person is no longer in the care of his or her parents and is at risk of harming him or herself or others.

There are several other agencies that may be able to offer help and support:

▷ for a young person who is at risk of harming other children or adults (police)
▷ where a young person has school attendance problems (Education Welfare Service)
▷ for a young person with suspected specific learning disability (school special-needs department)
▷ a young person with a substance misuse problem (local young persons' drug and alcohol services).

Voluntary organisations can often help children and adolescents with emotional or behavioural problems – for example the National Society for the Prevention of Cruelty to Children (NSPCC), local parental support groups (e.g. ADHD groups), and parenting groups run through programmes such as Sure Start.

Think ▷ *Has your practice got an up-to-date, local mental health resource directory?*

The GP curriculum can help us think about the different aspects to be taken into account when trying to help patients and families with what are usually very distressing conditions.

Primary care management

Primary care management includes the ability to balance looking for psychological illness whilst avoiding the habit of checking extensively for physical illness. We should aim to integrate ideas about the physical, psychological and social aspects into both the consultation and investigation of illness. Children experiencing mental health problems can be managed effectively in primary care, bearing in mind that several interventions may be needed for each mental health condition, including different forms of talking therapy, medication and self-help.

Psychotic illness as we have seen has a very low incidence in adolescents, but a general practice specialty registrar (GPStR) should familiarise him or herself with the varied ways that young people who are developing a first episode of psychosis might present. Similarly it is important to be able to describe early indicators of difficulty in the psychological wellbeing of children and young people, and respond quickly to concerns raised by parents, family members, early-years workers, teachers and others who are in close contact with the child or young person.

Person-centred care

It is important to be able to build rapport with children in difficulties, to be able to elicit a full history and understand the impact of the illness on the child and family. The aim is always to enable people experiencing mental health problems to be fully involved in decisions about their care, to be able to present them with choices as to which intervention may work best for them and to understand that this ability to choose improves the effectiveness of the intervention. Adolescence, already a turbulent time for some young people, is complicated by the handover to adult mental health services that can risk the continuity of care and stability of relationships. The GP can be an important focus at this time.

Specific problem-solving skills

As we have seen, several mental health conditions can be seen as extensions of a spectrum of normal behaviours. The art of primary care medicine is to be able to tease out those needing extra care or specialist intervention. Rapport building, history taking and observational skills will be needed.

A comprehensive approach

Managing educational and social issues as well as associated physical health problems of people with mental health problems is a specific primary care role.

Community orientation

The social circle of children and young people is focused on school. The implications of stigma and social exclusion can have extensive ramifications on the child's future life and career prospects. GPs need to know how to safeguard against the additional burden this can bring and challenge inequality.

Community orientation also involves working in partnership with other agencies to secure appropriate health and social interventions for individuals. It is also concerned with the wider public health of the local population and the ability of GPs to contribute to the development of specific services in the local health improvement programme.

A holistic approach

Social circumstances and family relationships can have a significant impact on mental illness and recovery may be contingent on the effective management of those social circumstances. Some aspects of mental illness are culturally determined and treatment and recovery depend on assumptions that may not be universal. Effective primary care management takes this context into account and works with cultural difference to ensure that diagnoses and treatment plans are acceptable to families. At times, folk treatments or actions within a community may not fit with the medical model and healthcare professionals need to be sensitive to this whilst at the same time ensuring the child or young person's safety and wellbeing are paramount.

References

1 • NHS Choices. *Autistic Spectrum Disorder*, www.nhsdirect.nhs.uk/articles/article.aspx?articleId=41 [accessed August 2009].

2 • Likierman H, Muter V. *ADHD (attention deficit hyperactivity disorder)*, www.netdoctor.co.uk/diseases/facts/adhd.htm [accessed August 2009].

3 • National Collaborating Centre for Mental Health, National Institute for Health and Clinical Excellence. *Clinical Guideline 72, Attention Deficit Hyperactivity Disorder: diagnosis and management of ADHD in children, young people and adults* London: The British Psychological Society, The Royal College of Psychiatrists, 2009, www.nice.org.uk/nicemedia/pdf/ADHDFullGuideline.pdf [accessed August 2009].

4 • Royal College of Psychiatrists. Factsheet 25: Suicide and attempted suicide. In: *Mental Health and Growing Up* (3rd edn) London: RCPsych. 2004, www.rcpsych.ac.uk/mentalhealthinfoforall/mentalhealthandgrowingup/25suicideandattempt.aspx [accessed August 2009].

5 • Royal College of Psychiatrists. Factsheet 24: Eating disorders in young people. In: *Mental Health and Growing Up* (3rd edn) London: RCPsych. 2004, www.rcpsych.ac.uk/mentalhealthinformation/mentalhealthandgrowingup/24.eatingdisordersinyoung.aspx [accessed August 2009].

6 • World Health Organization. *WHO Guide to Mental and Neurological Health in Primary Care* Geneva: WHO, www.mentalneurologicalprimarycare.org/page_view.asp?c=16&fc=002&did=2213 [accessed August 2009].

153

Dealing with disability

Mohammad Sawal

11

Introduction

This chapter looks at the special needs of children and families who are living with enduring, ongoing problems. We will see that a close relationship between health, social and educational services is vital to ensuring these children can reach their potential and take as active a role in society as possible. The importance of the primary care team is not only key in co-ordinating services but also in supporting all family members.

The following definitions are based on those of the World Health Organization.[1]

▷ **Impairment** ▶ is defined as loss or abnormality of psychological, physiological or anatomical structure or function.
▷ **Disability** ▶ is defined as the lack of ability (resulting from an impairment) to perform an activity that would normally be possible for a child of similar age. (This is sometimes referred to as 'activity limitation'.)
▷ **A handicap** ▶ is a disadvantage (resulting from an impairment/ disability) in fulfilling a role normal to that individual. (This is sometimes referred to as 'participation restriction'). Handicap is essentially 'social'.

Clearly there will be some overlap but, for example, we can see that a child who is blind (impairment) cannot read print books (disability) and therefore may not be able to attend a mainstream school (handicap).

Similarly a child with diplegia (spasticity of the legs, which is an impairment) may not be able to walk (disability) and therefore will not be able to play football with his or her peers (handicap).

The best practice guide for *Disabled Children and Young People and those with Complex Health Needs* sets out the following vision:[2]

We want to see:

▷ *Children and young people who are disabled or who have complex health needs, supported to participate in family and community activities and facilities.*

▷ *Health, education and social care services organised around the needs of children and young people and their families, with coordinated multi-agency assessments leading to prompt, convenient, responsive and high quality multi-agency interventions that maximise the child's ability to reach his or her full potential.*

▷ *Children and young people and their families actively involved in all decisions affecting them and shaping local services.*

Much of the care for any child with major disability will fall within the remit of community paediatric care and secondary or even tertiary care. The GP may be much less involved with diagnosis and delivery of care, but will have an important role within the multi-agency team, often being the first one approached with intercurrent problems. He or she will also have an overview of the wider family and may well have several members of the extended family on the list.

Causes of disability

We can divide the causes of disability into those that have their effects during pregnancy, those that occur around birth, and those that affect the child after birth.

Prenatal

▷ Genetic/chromosomal, infection (e.g. cytomegalovirus, rubella).
▷ Toxins, e.g. drugs such as sodium valproate.
▷ Placental insufficiency.

Perinatal

▷ Prematurity (leading to problems such as intraventricular haemorrhage, periventricular haemorrhage, periventricular leucomalacia).
▷ Infection.
▷ Meningitis.
▷ Toxins.
▷ Perinatal asphyxia.

Postnatal

▷ Such as infection, trauma (accidental or non-accidental), encephalopathy.

Whatever the cause of a disability it will usually become apparent as an abnormality in development. Thus it can be helpful to think of disabilities as:

▷ motor
▷ visual
▷ language
▷ social/behavioural.

Clearly children with severe disabilities may well have impairment in all areas. Other children will have impairment in only one of two of these areas. When dealing with the disabled child it is helpful to use a 'problem-based' approach.

The 'problem-based' approach

The child with disabilities is likely to have a number of handicaps. It is useful to work through the areas of their lives that may be affected. Clearly some areas will overlap. The list in Box 11.1 is designed to be used as a 'systems' approach. Rather than consider the cause of the handicap, we can use this approach to consider the way it affects the child. We can illustrate the systems-based approach by considering each of these and giving some examples.

Box 11.1 ○ **Systems-based approach to disability**

▷ Locomotor.
  ▶ Mobility.
  ▶ Posture.
▷ Neurology/developmental/manipulative skills.
  ▶ Vision.
  ▶ Hearing and language (including oral skills).
  ▶ Communication (verbal/nonverbal).
  ▶ Epilepsy.
▷ Social.
  ▶ Cognitive function and schooling.
  ▶ Financial support.
  ▶ Social support.
  ▶ Behaviour.
▷ Gastrointestinal.
▷ Growth.
▷ Respiratory.
▷ Cardiovascular.

Locomotor

Mobility

Physical impairments (e.g. cerebral palsy) frequently result in difficulties with standing and walking. Children with minor impairments may walk with the aid of special shoes or shoe inserts; moderate impairments may necessitate sticks while more severe impairment may confine the child to a wheelchair. Some children in wheelchairs may be able to move themselves through use of their arms and others by use of electric wheelchairs. Some children will be able to transfer from wheelchairs to, for example, the toilet or to bed while others will need help. Physical impairments often change with time. Children with low muscle tone are slow to achieve walking and when they do may tire easily, needing a wheelchair/pushchair for long distances. This is something that may improve with time. Some children with cerebral palsy may walk when young, but progress to needing a wheelchair when they reach a certain weight. Mobility can sometimes be maintained by physiotherapy (e.g. passive stretching, exercise regimens, night splinting or plastering), botulinum toxin injections or even surgery (osteotomy and tendon releases). Assessment of mobility is often carried out by a physiotherapist. In walking children gait analysis is sometimes used. Review by an orthopaedic surgeon is sometimes required.

Posture

Posture is often related to mobility. Children with physical disabilities often have difficulties standing or sitting; this affects their ability to interact with people and to use their fine motor skills. Special seating (often as part of wheelchairs) and standing frames may be useful. Splints or lycra suits are sometimes used to help with positioning. Assessment of posture is often carried out by occupational therapists. Children with lower-limb spasticity are prone to dislocated hips and spinal curvature. Regular review is required.

Fine motor/manipulative skills

Once posture is addressed the child may be in a more optimum position to use its fine motor skills. Special aids may be useful to help with day-to-day tasks: hand splints may help position the wrist in a more functional position; special utensils may help with eating; and using a keyboard may be easier than writing.

Vision

Children with handicap should always be assessed by specialist vision services.

Communication

The first investigation of any child with communication problems should be a hearing test. This is the commonest cause of language delay. If hearing is normal then there may be other reasons for communication problems. Language may simply be delayed or may be maldeveloped (e.g. autistic spectrum disorders). Children who have language delay are usually assessed and treated by a speech and language therapist. Children who are unable to communicate verbally may learn to sign using Makaton sign language for example.

Epilepsy

Thirty per cent of those with severe learning difficulties have epilepsy. Treatment can be difficult, with seizures sometime refractory to treatment. Simply administering medications to the child may be a challenge in itself.

Social

Schooling

Impairments lead to handicaps, which are by definition social. Some children with handicaps attend mainstream schools with support, while others attend special schools, many of which cater for children with specific problems. For any child with disability, a key intervention will be the statement of special educational needs. In order to find a school placement that best suits the individual child's needs, agreement should be reached between the parents and Local Education Authority. Following assessment by all professionals involved in the care of the child, a statement is drawn up specifying the placement and degree of support required. Mainstream schools will have a Special Educational Needs Co-ordinator (SENCO).

Financial support

Families of children with disabilities are entitled to financial support in the form of the Disability Living Allowance (DLA). Those with impaired mobility may also claim Mobility Allowance. Claims for allowances are usually facilitated by the child's social worker. Support can also be provided for necessary equipment such as wheelchairs and adaptations to the family home to help them look after the child at home. Adaptations to family homes are usually recommended after assessment by an occupational therapist. When not available from the local authority financial support can also be obtained from various charitable organisations.

Social support

In many cases this is provided by members of the extended family and friends. Some parents require periods away from their disabled child, perhaps to focus on the needs of other children, and respite care can be organised by social services for periods ranging from half a day to a fortnight holiday. Some families get to know regular foster carers for short-term respite.

Behaviour

Behaviour can sometimes be the most frustrating problem for parents. Children with special needs are a source of much tension, anxiety and worry within families. This can result in distortions in the usual relationships and a bending of the usual, expected behavioural norms. Children may 'get away' with more extremes of behaviour than their siblings, which can lead to jealousy and arguments, and escalation of problems in all the children in a family. Some problems are similar to those encountered by children without handicaps and the usual parenting advice can be given. Unfortunately, many are not amenable to treatment. Support from the Child and Adolescent Mental Health Services (CAMHS) may be beneficial.

Gastrointestinal

Maintaining adequate nutrition can be a problem for disabled children. Some may have difficulty swallowing, and drooling can be a significant problem. Limited swallowing or the risk of aspiration may necessitate insertion of a nasogastric tube or gastrostomy. The speech therapist may assess chewing and swallowing ability. Children with disabilities, like other children, require regular dental check-ups. These can require support from special dentists.

Toileting is often a problem for disabled children. Some have problems with continence, some with transfer to and from the toilet, and some have problems with soiling and wetting due to behaviour problems. Immobility may cause problems with constipation.

Growth

Certain conditions affect growth directly. It may also be impaired by poor nutrition. Children with poor mobility may become obese causing difficulties for carers.

Respiratory

Children with impaired gag reflexes are prone to aspiration and may develop recurrent pneumonias if oral feeding is continued. Children with more severe physical impairments may develop chest deformities that may impair respiration. Respiratory failure, usually precipitated by a pneumonia, is a common mode of death for children with more severe physical impairments.

Cardiovascular

Cardiovascular abnormalities are common in children with chromosomal causes of their disability (e.g. trisomy 21 – Down's syndrome).

Consider the following case of motor disability:

▶ The parents of Jack, a 17-month-old boy, come to see you. They are concerned that he is not walking yet. He is a bright little boy, sociable, but has few single words. He was born at 28 weeks' gestation and had a difficult neonatal course, requiring prolonged ventilatory support. You note that, although he can sit unsupported, he makes no attempt to pull to stand or cruise around the furniture.

The causes of delayed motor development are many, but there is a clue here in the prematurity and the early neonatal problems. One of the possibilities is cerebral palsy.

Cerebral palsy is defined as a permanent impairment of voluntary movement or posture, presumed to be due to permanent damage to the immature brain. The incidence of cerebral palsy is 1.7 to 3 cases per 1000 live births. It is a non-progressive impairment of motor function secondary to lesions in the developing brain. (This should be compared with handicaps due to progressive neurological conditions in which there is progressive loss of function.) Although cerebral palsy is non-progressive the impairment may change with time as the brain develops and the child grows. Lesions in the 'developing brain' refer to those occurring from the antenatal period up to the age of about 5 years (though some definitions put the cut-off at 2 years).

There are three main types of cerebral palsy:

▷ spastic cerebral palsy, which can be divided into diplegia (both legs), hemiplegia (both limbs on affected side) and quadriplegia (all limbs affected)
▷ ataxic cerebral palsy
▷ dyskinetic cerebral palsy.

Cerebral palsy classification is based on clinical description of neurological signs and history taking. Examination should be complete in order to ascertain all the features in Jack's story. Delayed walking, for example, could also be familial or, for boys, a rare disorder like Duchenne muscular dystrophy.

The key step will be a multidisciplinary assessment and involvement of other professionals to see how pervasive the difficulties are. The key professionals involved will be the:

▷ **physiotherapist** ▶ responsible for assessment and support for development of motor skills
▷ **speech and language therapist** ▶ help in feeding, communication and speech assessment
▷ **occupational therapist** ▶ assessment of fine motor skills, the need for equipment that helps in different aspects of daily living such as toileting, seating, feeding, etc. They also help to assess different adaptations that are required to be made at home according to the need of the child.

The early-years team and portage is a home-visiting educational service for pre-school children. These team members support the family, assess the child's needs and provide appropriate support such as arranging placement in nursery and later assess the educational need of the child.

As months go by, Jack should also be assessed for specific associated problems.

Feeding difficulties

Children with cerebral palsy can suffer from gastro-oesophageal reflux and have gastro-oesophagitis. It is important to address positioning and consistency of food, and consider the need for gastrostomy feeding.

162

Drooling

This can be a problem when motor difficulties make swallowing inefficient. It can be treated by attention to positioning, exercise and medication such as glycopyrronium or hyoscine patches. In severe cases treatment may be by botulinum injection in submandibular glands and surgical procedures like duct ligation, rerouting and removal of salivary glands.

Dislocated hip

This can result from poor posture. Seating management can help to prevent dislocation.

Bowel and bladder problems

Incontinence and constipation may result from learning difficulties or with immobility of the child. Good routines need to be established; parents may need an explanation about normal bowel function and giving dietary advice.

Vision problems

Vision problems are common, particularly myopia, cortical vision impairment and squint, and will need formal assessment.

Hearing problems

This can occur in up to 20–30 per cent of children with cerebral palsy, particularly sensorineural deafness. It requires assessment.

Epilepsy

Around 21 per cent of children with cerebral palsy develop epilepsy, which may be difficult to control.

Psychological problems

These may be related to physical disability or underlying brain disorder, but also arise from the long-term effects of living with a disabling condition. As time goes by Jack's needs will change and, especially, transition care during the move to adult services will be vital.

Educational issues

Cerebral palsy is a physical disability. Most children will go to mainstream school with support and specific adaptations at school, such as wheelchair access and computer or writing aids.

General and specific learning difficulties

General learning difficulties tend to be related to physical problems. However, Jack may have specific learning difficulties in certain areas and as he gets older he will need a formal assessment.

Further specific treatment

Cerebral palsy is often complicated by spasticity of the limbs, which is a velocity-dependent increase in resistance to passive stretch. This can be treated with oral medication like baclofen, which is an analogue of gamma-aminobutyric acid (GABA), or botulinum toxin, which inhibits the release of neurotransmitter acetylcholine at the neuromuscular junction. Surgical procedures are sometimes used to aid mobility and posture. Tendons can be lengthened to relieve contracture or can be transplanted to achieve a better function.

Consider Ryan, who has a communication problem.

▶ Ryan is two and a half and his parents bring him to you with concerns about his speech and language development. He can only say a few single words, although he has achieved his motor milestones and has no significant past medical history.

Communication and speech and language are highly developed human skills. Understanding speech and sound production involves a large part of the brain. Approximately 5 per cent of the children at school entry have been recorded to have unintelligible speech. The majority of these children have added emotional and behaviour problems.

The first step is to exclude hearing impairment. The assessment of these children requires a detailed history and a general developmental assessment, including hearing assessment. A careful history may also uncover specific problems like feeding difficulties, problems with chewing, dribbling or difficulties with social relationships.

The assessment of speech and language is a specialised job done by experienced therapists. Assessment looks at the different components of speech,

such as attention and control, comprehension, expressive speech, phrenol-
ogy, oral facial skills and semantic and pragmatic assessment that includes
understanding the meaning of words and context of language. Ryan will be
assessed for nonverbal communication that includes tone of the voice, body
posture, facial expression and gestures. Children who have communication
and social interaction problems associated also with a ritualised activity
should be assessed for autistic spectrum disorder.

The management of children such as Ryan is predominantly by a speech and
language therapist, who advises the parents, nursery and school how to help
language development. The multidisciplinary team also monitor these young
children and work with them either in groups or on an individual basis.

Two phrases might be applied to Ryan. *Developmental delay* tends to be
used below the age of 5 years (pre-school) and may pertain to delay in any
of the four main areas of development (gross motor, fine motor and vision,
hearing and language, and social). Multidisciplinary assessment may be
necessary to map the extent of the delay in each field. This leads on to multidisciplinary intervention.

Learning difficulties tends to be used in school-aged children (5 and above).
By this age associated impairments are often more clearly defined (e.g. spastic diplegia, ataxia, autism, etc.). Learning difficulties are usually assessed
by an educational psychologist and/or a teacher and an educational plan
devised in the form of a 'statement of special educational needs'. Learning
difficulties can be expressed in terms of IQ or, more usually, 'developmental
quotient' (<50 severe, 50–75 moderate to mild – the median IQ of the population is approximately 95). However, development/ability is probably more
usefully expressed in terms of functional ability (i.e. at 10 years of age Ryan
may perform to the standard of a 6-year-old).

Children with specific or global learning difficulties may become subject
to a common assessment framework (CAF), which is a multidisciplinary
assessment to ensure children receive the co-ordinated package of care they
require. This may well take place at a child development centre, where community paediatricians are often based with other community professionals.
These act as a resource for assessment and management of children with
disabilities, usually those under 5 years' old. Older children are usually followed routinely in school by the school medical service.

Further reading

▷ Children's Workforce Development Council. *Common Assessment
Framework for Children and Young People* Leeds: CWDC, 2007.

165

▷ Crysdale W S, Raveh E, McCann C, *et al.* Management of drooling in individuals with neurodisability: a surgical experience *Development Medicine and Child Neurology* 2001; **43**: 379–83.

▷ Disability Living Allowance. www.direct.gov.uk/en/DisabledPeople/ index.htm [accessed August 2009].

▷ Jongerius P H, Rotteveel J J, van den Hoogen F, *et al.* Botulinum toxin A: a new option for the treatment of drooling in children with cerebral palsy *European Journal of Pediatrics* 2001; **160(8)**: 509–12.

▷ Merton Council, Education, Leisure and Libraries. *Achievement and Inclusion: Merton's policy & strategy on special educational needs 2005–2008* London: Merton Council, 2005, www.merton.gov.uk/learning/ edinclusion/edspecialneeds/sen_policy_2005.pdf [accessed August 2009].

References

1 • World Health Organization. *Classification of Impairments, Disabilities and Handicaps* (ICIDH) Geneva: WHO, 2001.

2 • Department of Health, Department for Education and Skills. *National Service Framework for Children, Young People and Maternity Services: disabled children and young people and those with complex health needs* London: DoH, 2004, www.dh.gov.uk/en/ Publicationsandstatistics/Publications/PublicationsPolicyAndGuidance/DH_4089112 [accessed August 2009].

Important themes in child and adolescent health

12

Moli Paul

Introduction

What do I need to learn in this area?

This chapter aims to describe what is meant by concepts such as confidentiality and consent, Gillick competence and parental responsibility. We will consider children and young people with special needs or in special circumstances and how issues such as the rights of and duties owed to children and young people impact on our practice.

Overview

Legal advice, service provision and policy terminology often differs in relation to children and young people compared with adults. Whilst thinking about and interacting with them as individuals, GPs simultaneously should understand children and young people in the context of their families and communities, supporting their parents and carers who are supporting and protecting them. GPs should respond to their developmental needs and specific vulnerabilities whilst respecting them, promoting and recognising their participatory rights, whether they are competent to consent or not. A duty of care is clearly owed to children that means GPs should practise within the law and always act in the best interests of the child.

Terminology

GPs often use terminology in relation to groups of children and should be clear about its meaning.

CHILDREN IN SPECIAL CIRCUMSTANCES

This refers to groups who traditionally have found it difficult to access services because they get 'lost', either from universal or specialist health, social care or educational services, or between agencies. They include 'Looked After Children', care leavers, the homeless or those exposed to domestic violence. An example is a child of substance-misusing parents, who is not brought to health professionals when unwell. Another is a Looked After Child, moving between foster homes, who never receives locality-based specialist health care. They are at risk of doing worse in life than their peers and GPs should co-operate with different services to help them.[1]

SPECIAL NEEDS

In health services, the term 'children with special needs' tends to be used in relation to disabled children and young people, and those with complex health needs. This includes those with learning disabilities, autism spectrum disorders, sensory and/or physical impairments and emotional and/or behavioural disorders. Not all disabled children need health interventions but others will need ongoing, co-ordinated care from their families and friends, and a number of professionals and agencies.[2] Some may also be considered children in special circumstances.

The social care definition of a 'child in need' applies to those unlikely to achieve or maintain 'a reasonable standard of health or development' or whose 'health or development is likely to be significantly impaired' without the provision of additional services.[3] These include: those who have suffered significant harm or who are parentless (e.g. orphans and unaccompanied asylum seekers); whose families are in acute difficulty (e.g. homelessness) or are significantly dysfunctional (e.g. domestic violence, family breakdown); who have physical, sensory, learning or emotional and behavioural disabilities; who are young carers of parents with physical or mental health problems; whose behaviour is socially unacceptable (e.g. young offenders); or who live in low-income families or independently. In education services those with special educational needs include children and young people with specific or general learning difficulties or social, emotional and behavioural difficulties.[4]

Communication

The basis for providing good care is effective communication, i.e. establishing 'what children, young people and their parents want and need to know, what issues are important to them, and what opinions or fears they have about their health or treatment'.[5] This includes:

1 ▷ Involving children and young people in discussions about their care

2 ▷ Being honest and open with them and their parents, while respecting confidentiality

3 ▷ Listening to and respecting their views about their health, and responding to their concerns and preferences

4 ▷ Explaining things using language or other forms of communication they can understand

5 ▷ Considering nonverbal communication and the effect of surroundings in which to meet

6 ▷ Giving them opportunities to ask questions, and answering these honestly and to the best of your ability

7 ▷ Doing all you can to make open and truthful discussion possible, including involving parents or other people, and also seeing children alone, as necessary

8 ▷ Giving them the same time and respect given to adult patients.[5]

GPs should give children and young people information about their conditions or difficulties, what any proposed investigations or treatments involve, how likely interventions are to succeed and the risks entailed by different options, including no treatment. Also, GPs should explain who will be involved in their care and that they are entitled to change their minds. Good timing, digestible chunks of information, and checking they have understood key points, e.g. by asking them to explain things back, are useful.[5]

Making clear to children and young people that they have rights to participate in decision-making,[6] unless they choose to defer to their parents or carers, is important and GPs can indicate that their views, values and preferences are taken seriously. By encouraging and supporting them to be active, informed decision-makers, GPs can nurture their abilities to take responsibility for their own health, emotional and social development and wellbeing, in the present, the future and into adulthood.[1] These targets can only be achieved if GPs have child- and young person-friendly communication and consultation skills.

A wider view of communicating involves ensuring that healthcare premises are child- or teenager-friendly.[7] This includes being explicit about consent and confidentiality policies at surgeries and within consultations. If GPs value and take into account children's views in the planning, delivery and evaluation of services, they should ask them rather than make assumptions.[1]

Communicating and decision-making with families

Communicating with families is a skill in itself. It involves paying attention to individuals and the group at the same time, facilitating everyone having a voice, regardless of age, developmental level, relationship or power differentials, providing information and then, perhaps, making decisions. Each can participate at four different levels of decision-making: being informed, expressing a view, influencing decision-making and being the main decision-maker.[8] At times, communication may be facilitated by seeing children or young people and their parents separately and together. We should aim to reach consensus[9] or concordance, and this can usually be reached. However, if not possible, we should consider issues such as confidentiality, consent and refusal.

Confidentiality

Confidentiality applies when one person discloses information (in verbal, written or electronic form) to someone else in special circumstances (e.g. within the doctor–patient relationship), where it is reasonable to expect that the information will not be shared without permission. There are some important limits (e.g. for child protection reasons), which we should be clear about. Practically, we might start consultations with children and young people by saying:

I will not tell anyone what you tell me without asking you first. This is called confidentiality. Sometimes it is useful to share what we have talked about, for instance with your parents, so they can help you. If you really do not want someone else to know, please tell me. Please remember though that if I think you, or someone else, is in danger, I might have to share what we have talked about, to keep people safe. I will always try to talk to you first, if this needs to happen.

Our duty to maintain confidentiality exists whether our patients expect it or not. Clarity about the scope and limits of confidentiality helps, especially with teenagers, and particularly when we discuss sensitive issues such as sexual health, contraception[10] and drug and alcohol use.[11] Confidentiality is a legal duty but also a professional[12,5] and employment-related[13] obligation. We have the same duty of confidentiality to children and young people as to adults.

Sharing information

Children and young people may be happy for information to be shared with their parents and vice versa. If a competent child or young person does not want to share information, we should encourage them otherwise, justifying our request; however, if they insist, we should respect their views.[5,9]

One exception is when there is serious risk to the health, safety or welfare of any child or young person. We should then follow national information-sharing guidance[14] and locally agreed child protection protocols.[15] Other exceptions include our duties to protect the public (e.g. from acts of terrorism,[16] communicable diseases[12] or unfit drivers[12]), the patient in life-threatening situations (e.g. where a suicide attempt is suspected), other service providers in life-threatening situations and when directed by a court.[5,12] We also have the power, but not a duty, to disclose information to prevent or detect a crime.[17]

When considering information-sharing, whether we break confidentiality or not, we should document the harm we are seeking to avoid, what the disclosure is intended to achieve and any benefits to the young person's well-being.[12] The information should be accurate, up to date, necessary for the intended purpose and only shared securely with those who need to know.[14] Unless to do so would compromise safety, we should make disclosures to third parties such as parents, police or social services only after discussing the need for this with the young person and offering to help him or her tell the relevant person or agency themselves. Although the competence of the young person is an important consideration, we should generally follow the same rules if considering breaking the confidence of young people who lack competence. When in doubt, we should seek advice.[14]

Access to medical records

Children and young people with capacity and their parents, and the parents of those lacking capacity, all have legal rights to view the young person's health records. In Scotland, those aged 12 years or over are legally presumed to be competent to access their own health records. We should not, however, disclose information that would cause serious harm or information about other people, who have not consented to such disclosure.[5]

Consent

Giving consent is a specific sort of decision-making and permission-giving. The law and guidance constantly change, so we need to keep up to date.[18] When dealing with children and young people, we should bear in mind age-related differences in the law,[19,20] National Health Service requirements[1] and professional advice.[5,9]

Consent should be given voluntarily by an appropriately informed person (the patient or where relevant someone with parental responsibility for a patient under the age of 18) who has the capacity to consent to the intervention in question. Acquiescence where the person does not know what the intervention entails is not 'consent'.[19] There are three traditional aspects of consent: capacity, information and voluntariness. With children, it can be useful to add a fourth: decision-making.

Decision-making and voluntariness

It is useful to establish whether a child or young person is an active decision-maker. We can encourage those who are not by informing them and their parents of their rights (see below) and encouraging participation. It is also important to establish who is the main decision-maker (e.g. where more than one person's consent would be acceptable (see below)) or where, regardless of who can consent, the child's wishes or preferences should be respected (e.g. when coercion would be too harmful, undermine the intended outcome or impair family or therapeutic relationships[21]).

Information

We should provide information in developmentally appropriate language and formats. We should also ask children and young people what information they want, as our predictions about what is important to them may be incorrect.

Capacity, Gillick competence and Fraser guidelines

The terms capacity and competence are sometimes used interchangeably. In English and Welsh law, however, capacity is used in relation to those 16 years and older,[22] whereas Gillick competence is used in relation to under 16-year-olds.[23]

Capacity requires that a person understands information about the decision, retains that information, uses or weighs the information as part of the decision-making process, and communicates his or her decision by any means.[24] Capacity can change over time and a person may contemporaneously lack capacity to make one decision but not another.[25]

To be Gillick competent, an under-16 needs to have 'a sufficient understanding and intelligence to be capable in making up his mind on the matter requiring decision'.[23] If a child or young person refuses life-saving treatment or makes decisions that could seriously undermine his or her health, the courts sometimes require more from him or her, e.g. to choose wisely and in his or her best interests,[26] demonstrate stability of choice[27] or even have a full understanding of choosing to die.[28]

Sometimes Gillick competence is referred to as Fraser competence. It is more correct to use Gillick competence as the test by which to judge competence in the under-16s in relation to healthcare decisions in general and limit the use of 'Fraser guidelines' to the summary of Lord Fraser's judgement on the provision of contraceptive advice to under-16s, especially without the explicit consent of their parents[29] (see Table 12.1).

Table 12.1 ○ *Gillick competence and Fraser guidelines*

	Gillick competence	Fraser guidelines
Application	Judging competence in the under-16s in relation to healthcare decisions in general	The provision of contraceptive advice to the under-16s
Requirements for competence to consent	To have sufficient understanding and intelligence to be capable in making up his or her mind on the matter requiring decision[23]	The young person understands the doctor's advice
		The doctor cannot persuade the young person to inform his or her parents or allow the doctor to inform the parents that he or she is seeking contraceptive advice
		The young person is very likely to begin or continue having sexual intercourse with or without contraceptive treatment
		The young person's physical or mental health or both are likely to deteriorate if he or she does not receive contraceptive advice or treatment
		The young person's best interests require the doctor to give contraceptive advice or treatment, or both, without parent consent[30]

Giving and refusing consent

Essentially, any of the following *can* give consent: 16–17-year-olds who have capacity, *Gillick-competent* minors, a person or local authority with parental responsibility, a court, or a person caring for the child (but only when reasonable in the circumstances and necessary to promote or safeguard the child's welfare).[20] We should usually respect a competent minor's refusal.[5,9,20] If he or she refuses life-saving treatment or makes decisions that could seriously undermine his or her health, and we have consent from a person with parental responsibility, we should consider the minor's best interests, balancing the harms associated with overriding his or her refusal with the benefits of treatment. If there is irresolvable disagreement about best interests, we should consult some or all of the following: members of the multidisciplinary team, professional peers, professional and organisational managers, the named or designated doctor for child protection or an independent advocate.[5] We should seek legal advice, from a medical protection organisation or our NHS Trust's legal advisers, if necessary, and especially if considering applying to the court.

Community assessment and treatment of under-18-year-olds for mental health problems entails similar reasoning. On infrequent occasions when a child or young person needs admission to a mental health hospital, we should consider a range of legislation [22,31-33] and associated guidance,[34] and discuss with specialist mental health professionals.

The legal concept of 'parental responsibility'

Parents are the main people with responsibility for bringing up their children and the state should help parents with this parental responsibility (PR),[1,32] which is defined as all the rights, duties, power and authority that a parent has in relation to his or her child, flowing from duties towards the child and not from the adult's status as a parent. Parental duties include caring for the child and raising the child to be morally, physically and emotionally healthy.[35] Most but not all biological parents have PR, others can legally have PR, and it can be held by more than one person/authority (see Table 12.2).

We should remember that parents without PR nonetheless may play an essential role in their children's lives and should generally be included in discussions about their children's health.[36]

Parental responsibility and consent

Anyone with PR can legally consent to treatment on behalf of the child or young person under 18 years. Where more than one person holds PR, consent is only required from one of them, or the child or young person if competent to consent. However, we should always seek to reach consensus. If this is not possible, we could proceed with one person's consent, acting in

Table 12.2 ○ *Who has parental responsibility (PR)?* [37]

	Biological parents	Others
Automatic	▷ Biological mothers ▷ Biological fathers If named on the birth certificate for children born after 1 December 2003 in England and Wales, after 15 April 2002 in Northern Ireland, and after 4 May 2006 in Scotland Of children born before these dates, only if the father was married to the mother at the time of the child's conception, or at birth, or at some time after the child's birth	
Acquired	▷ Biological father without PR ▶ by Parental Responsibility Agreement with the mother, or ▶ Parental Responsibility Order through the courts	▷ Someone appointed as a guardian or on the order of a court ▷ Adoptive parents on legal adoption ▷ Married step-parents or civil partners through ▶ a Parental Responsibility Agreement with the mother, or ▶ a Parental Responsibility Order through the courts ▷ The High Court's inherent jurisdiction in relation to minors (children and young people under 18 years of age): ▶ *parens patriae*, derived from the parental jurisdiction of the Crown to which all British children are potentially subject ▶ wardship proceedings
Lost/restricted	▷ Restriction can only occur by court order ▷ Lost if the child is adopted	▷ Restriction can only occur by court order
Not lost	▷ Following divorce ▷ If the child is in care or custody	

175

the best interests of the child, unless the disagreement is over a controversial or elective intervention. In such cases we should seek legal advice.

If a parent or carer who does not hold PR seeks treatment for a child, we should seek the views of someone with PR. If we believe people with PR are not making decisions in the best interests of the child, we may need to follow local safeguarding children procedures [15] or court review. If emergency treatment, i.e. treatment necessary to preserve life or prevent serious deterioration, is required, we may need to proceed whilst seeking judicial review. However, we should not give non-emergency treatment in the interim.[5,9]

The rights of both the parent and the child or young person in the family

Children and young people's rights

Children and young people have a number of legal, sociocultural and moral rights, which we should balance with each other and the rights of other people such as their parents.[38] Their legal rights result from health care, child and family and common law as well as international conventions such as the United Nations *Convention on the Rights of the Child*.[6] We should consider all our roles at any meeting with children and young people, as each may entail rights and duties (see case study). We have duties to support children to be healthy, stay safe, enjoy and achieve, make a positive contribution to society and achieve economic wellbeing.[1] They have rights to protection, provision and participation,[6] and we should balance their basic (e.g. safety, sustenance and shelter), developmental (i.e. maximising potential) and choice-based interests or needs.[5,9,39]

Parents' rights

Parents and carers have rights to information, access to appropriate services and support, so they can help and care for their children, keeping them safe and healthy and providing them with the best possible chances in life.[1,5,6,32] Parents also have rights as individuals[37] and the duties we owe them will depend on which of the above rights are relevant in any given scenario. In relation to the same family, these duties may differ over time, especially as the child matures and gains competence.

The balance between the rights of parents and their children

The family is generally accepted as the best environment within which to bring up children.[1,6,32] Usually, parents will know their children best and want the best for their children. Sometimes, though, there may be real or potential conflicts between what is best for the child and what their parents want or need for themselves. Parents may be abusive towards or neglectful of a child. Problems, such as substance misuse, severe chronic or short-term physical or mental health problems, or social or interpersonal issues (such as severe poverty or domestic violence), can limit their ability to respond to their children's needs. All doctors have child protection duties.[1,5] Whilst we should support such parents with their special needs, we must prioritise the safeguarding of children and young people, whether they or their parents are our patients.[15] In these cases, work with other professionals and agencies, especially health visitors and social services, may be necessary to assess children's needs and their parents' capacity.

How does the RCGP curriculum help us to consider issues in this area?

Primary care management

▷ Communication can be facilitated by seeing children with parents/carers and young people by themselves, but also vice versa at times.

▷ Multi-agency working is important, especially in relation to safeguarding children and young people and those in special circumstances, or who have special needs.

▷ Ensure children and their parents/carers have developmentally appropriate information so that they can make decisions about their health and wellbeing.

▷ Help parents with problems, including substance misuse, domestic violence and physical or mental health problems, but always consider the wellbeing of, and safeguard, their children.

Person-centred care

▷ Developmentally appropriate communication with children and young people is key.

▷ We should listen to them and involve them in their own care, alongside their parents and carers, taking into account their increasing maturity, and balancing the need for confidentiality with their parents' need for information. The aim should be to reach consensus or concordance.

▷ We should support parents with caring for their children by providing adequate information, support and access to services.

Specific problem-solving skills

▷ Have a thorough understanding of development and its relevance to communication and decision-making.
▷ Understand that children may be dependent on carers to access health care and that missed appointments should raise concern.

A comprehensive approach

▷ Assess the developmental needs of children and young people in the context of their families, including their parents' capacity to care for them and their parents' own special needs. Recognise that some may need referral for multi-agency assessment and/or support.
▷ Understand the vulnerabilities of those in need and in special circumstances. Respond to their needs, including through referral and joint working.
▷ Describe the issues involved in delivering services for young people relating to access, communication, confidentiality and consent.[7]
▷ Follow the revised guidance around the provision of contraception to under-16s, including issues around confidentiality.[10]

Community orientation

▷ Understand care pathways and local systems of care for children, including the meaning of terminology and the law.

A holistic approach

▷ Maximise the understanding of children and young people about their rights.
▷ Describe their needs and interests, especially in order to balance them and act in their best interests.

Attitudinal aspects

Describe the importance of:

▷ treating children and young people equitably, and with respect for their beliefs, preferences, dignity and rights
▷ issues of confidentiality and consent
▷ record-keeping and sharing information.

Case history

Consider the following. Kayleigh is a 15-year-old female who has 'heart-burn'. She attends surgery alone. Dr Smith has previously only seen her with her mother. He starts by asking about symptoms. Through discussion, he suspects she has uncomplicated dyspepsia but discovers she has been eating irregularly, and drinking significant amounts of alcohol most nights in the company of her mother. Kayleigh says she is worried that her mother is 'depressed' following a recent 'break-up', drinking constantly and unable to shop or cook. Kayleigh keeps her company, but has no money and, anyway, cannot cook. She has no other family support. Dr Smith tries to ask more about Kayleigh's mother but she replies, 'I don't want to get Mum into trouble. You can't say anything, you know. I've got rights. Confidentiality – that's what it's called, isn't it? Can you give me something for my heartburn?'

Questions

1 ▷ *What are the main issues?*
2 ▷ *What should Dr Smith do?*
3 ▷ *How could the consultation have been managed differently?*

Suggestions

1 ▷ *What are the main issues?*
   ▶ Confidentiality.
   ▶ Treatment, consent and competence.
   ▶ Safeguarding young people, supporting parents with problems and meeting the needs of a young person in special circumstances.

2 ▷ *What should Dr Smith do?*
   ▶ Acknowledge rights to confidentiality but indicate the exceptions to these.
   ▶ Assess whether Kayleigh is Gillick competent (as she is under 16 years of age).
   ▶ Encourage her to have a joint consultation with her mother the following day. One aim is to seek consensus between the young person, person with parental responsibility and doctor, regarding treatment and seeking consent. The second is to facilitate discussion about sharing information in order to start a multi-agency package of assessment and care to meet the

needs of both mother and child, to assess parenting capacity and investigate any child abuse or neglect. The latter should address the needs of Kayleigh as a young person in special circumstances.

▶ If Kayleigh refuses further consultation with her mother but wants treatment, Dr Smith should assess her competence to consent, and provide treatment if necessary. He should also explain that he will have to share the information with social services so that they can assess her safety and wellbeing, and arrange for help and support if necessary. He should offer to see her again or establish what other professionals she might trust.

3 ▷ *How could the consultation have been managed differently?*

▶ If the surgery had clear information about young people and confidentiality, Kayleigh might have known the exceptions to confidentiality.

▶ Dr Smith, noting that this is the first time he has seen Kayleigh alone, could have taken the opportunity to discuss consent and confidentiality issues at the beginning of the consultation.

References

1 • Department Of Health. *National Service Framework for Children, Young People and Maternity Services: core standards* London: DoH, 2004.

2 • Department Of Health. *National Service Framework for Children, Young People and Maternity Services: standard 8: disabled children and young people and those with complex health needs* London: DoH, 2004.

3 • Children Act 1989, Section 17(10).

4 • DirectGov. *What are Special Educational Needs?* www.direct.gov.uk/en/Parents/Schoolslearninganddevelopment/SpecialEducationalNeeds/DG_4008600 [accessed August 2009].

5 • General Medical Council. *0–18 years: guidance for all doctors* London: GMC, 2007.

6 • UNICEF. *Convention on the Rights of the Child*, www.unicef.org/crc/index_30160.html [accessed August 2009].

7 • Royal College of Nursing, Royal College of General Practitioners. *Getting it Right for Teenagers in Your Practice* London: RCGP, 2002, www.rcn.org.uk/__data/assets/pdf_file/0008/78542/001798.pdf [accessed August 2009].

8 • Alderson P, Montgomery J. *Health Care Choices: making decisions with children* London: Institute for Public Policy Research, 1996.

9 • British Medical Association. *Consent, Rights and Choices in Health Care for Children and Young People* London: BMA, 2001.

10 • Department of Health. *Best Practice Guidance for Doctors and other Health Professionals on the Provision of Advice and Treatment to Young People under 16 on Contraception, Sexual and Reproductive Health* London: DoH, 2004, www.dh.gov.uk/prod_consum_dh/groups/dh_digitalassets/@dh/@en/documents/digitalasset/dh_4086914.pdf [accessed August 2009].

11 • DrugScope, Alcohol Concern. *Drugs: guidance for the youth service* London: DrugScope, 2006, www.drugscope.org.uk/Resources/Drugscope/Documents/PDF/Education%20and%20Prevention/drugsguideservice.pdf [accessed August 2009].

12 • General Medical Council. *Confidentiality: protecting and providing information* London: GMC, 2004.

13 • Department of Health. *Confidentiality: NHS code of practice* London: DoH, 2003.

14 • Department for Education and Skills. *Information Sharing: practitioner's guide – integrated working to improve outcomes for children and young people* London: DfES, 2006, www.ecm.gov.uk/informationsharing [accessed August 2009].

15 • Her Majesty's Government. *Working Together to Safeguard Children: a guide to inter-agency working to safeguard and promote the welfare of children* London: TSO, 2006.

16 • Prevention of Terrorism Act 1971.

17 • Crime and Disorder Act 1998, Section 115.

18 • Department of Health. Consent key documents, www.dh.gov.uk/en/Publichealth/Scientificdevelopmentgeneticsandbioethics/Consent/Consentgeneralinformation/index.htm [accessed August 2009].

19 • Department of Health. *Reference Guide to Consent for Examination or Treatment* London: DoH, 2001, www.dh.gov.uk/en/Publicationsandstatistics/Publications/PublicationsPolicyAndGuidance/DH_4006757 [accessed August 2009].

20 • Department of Health. *Seeking Consent: working with children* London: DoH, 2001, www.dh.gov.uk/en/Publicationsandstatistics/Publications/PublicationsPolicyAndGuidance/DH_4007005 [accessed August 2009].

21 • Paul M, Newns K, Creedy K V. Some ethical issues that arise from working with families in the National Health Service *Clinical Ethics* 2006; **1(2)**: 76–81.

22 • Mental Capacity Act 2005.

23 • Gillick v West Norfolk and Wisbech Area Health Authority [1986] A.C.112.

24 • Mental Capacity Act 2005, Section 3(1).

25 • Ministry of Justice. *Mental Capacity Act 2005 Code of Practice* London: TSO, 2007, www.justice.gov.uk/docs/mca-cp.pdf [accessed August 2009].

26 • Gillick v West Norfolk and Wisbech Area Health Authority [1985] 3 All ER 402HL.

27 • Re R [1991].

28 • Re E [1993].

29 • Wheeler R. Gillick or Fraser? A plea for consistency over competence in children *British Medical Journal* 2006; **332**: 807.

30 • Gillick v West Norfolk and Wisbech Area Health Authority [1985] 3 All ER 402HL.

31 • Mental Health Acts 1983/2007.

32 • Children Act 1989.

33 • Human Rights Act 1998.

34 • Department of Health. *Mental Health Act 1983 Code of Practice* London: DoH, 2008.

35 • Children Act 1989, Section 3(1).

36 • Human Rights Act 1998, Article 8.

37 • Ethics Department of the British Medical Association. *Parental Responsibility: guidance from the British Medical Association* London: BMA, 2008, www.bma.org.uk/ethics/consent_ and_capacity/Parental.jsp [accessed August 2009].

38 • Paul M. Rights *Archives of Disease in Childhood* 2007; **92(8)**: 720–5.

39 • Eekelaar J. Parents and children: rights, responsibilities and needs *Adoption and Fostering* 1983; **7**: 7–10.

Sexual health of young people

13

Joyce Williams

Introduction

The median age for first sexual intercourse in the UK fell during the 1990s to around 16 years, for both boys and girls. The UK teenage pregnancy rate is amongst the highest in Europe. This chapter looks at the sexual health needs of this group, those thinking of becoming sexually active and those at risk from unwanted sexual activity.

The previous difference observed between the sexes, that boys were generally older at age of first intercourse, has now disappeared. About 18 per cent of boys and 15 per cent of girls report having had full sexual intercourse prior to the age of 15, with similar proportions reporting experience of oral sex.[1] Giving sexual health advice to teenagers is different from giving contraceptive advice to adults because of the typical characteristics of the teenage population, and their requirements. Studies have shown that confidentiality is a particularly important issue for this population, as well as ease of access to services.[2]

To be seen and treated alone, i.e. without a suitable adult present, girls under the age of 16 have to be assessed as Fraser (or Gillick) competent. This is further discussed in Chapter 12 but, in summary, this means:

▷ they must be able to understand the effect that their actions may have on their health (that if they have sex they may become pregnant)
▷ they must be able to understand the effects that the treatment (contraception) would have on their health, including side effects
▷ they must be at risk of harm if no action were taken (i.e. having, or about to have, a sexually active relationship)
▷ the involvement of an adult, not necessarily a parent, but perhaps an older sister, cousin or friend – someone that they trust – has been discussed with them but they have chosen not to involve the adult
▷ the doctor or nurse must consider that they are acting in the best interests of the girl.[3]

If all these criteria appear to be met, the girl may be judged to be competent to consent to a sexual relationship and to decisions about contraception without the involvement of an adult.[4]

We also have a responsibility to make some basic assessment of the nature of the sexual relationship. For example, a 15-year-old girl with a 16-year-old boyfriend, in the year above her at school, appears to represent a more evenly balanced relationship than that of a 15-year-old girl and a 25-year-old man, especially if there is also a difference in 'power status' between them or a child protection issue (e.g. she sings in the choir and he is the choir master). Any suspected risk of coercion or undue influence, or even of the girl putting herself in a position where she may stand to gain from the relationship, should be explored in detail (e.g. she may be given a solo if she has sex with the choir master). A vulnerable teenage girl with suspected coercion into a sexual relationship would be a justifiable reason for breaking the girl's confidentiality and involving the local child protection team.

Contraception

Encouraging girls to access contraception and to adhere to medication regimes can be difficult. In the UK, the most popular contraceptive method among teenage girls is the combined pill. Long-acting contraceptives (LARCs) are relatively under-used in teenagers in the UK compared with other countries.

One of the barriers to uptake of contraception might be information about success and failure rates. Figure 13.1 shows the contraceptive failure rates of various methods in the first year of use, but we should bear in mind the data are for women of all ages.[5] Norplant is no longer available in the UK but has been replaced by Implanon, which has a similar extremely low failure rate.

The combined oral contraceptive pill

The combined oral contraceptive pill (COCP) contains oestrogen and hence is associated with small risks of deep vein thrombosis (DVT) and stroke. However, it offers the advantage of providing the taker with some degree of control over her menstrual cycle, as well as being a reliable form of contraception. For teenage girls, control over their periods is an important issue, whereas the risk of something happening to them at some time in the future is easy to ignore. The risks of DVT or stroke are actually very low for fit and active teenage girls, especially if they do not smoke. The risks increase with factors like obesity, smoking and lack of exercise. Sadly, these risk factors are becoming more common in our teenage population.

There is also an increased risk of stroke with the COCP in migraine sufferers, if the migraine is associated with an aura. Migraine often begins

Figure 13.1 ○ *Contraceptive failure rates*

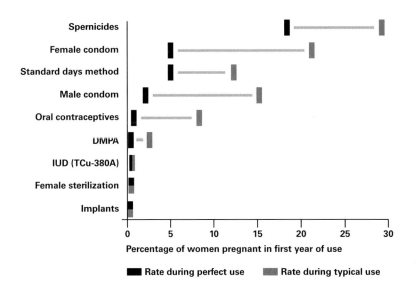

Percentage of women pregnant in first year of use

■ Rate during perfect use   ▨ Rate during typical use

Source: Family Health International. http://fhi.org/training/en/modules/FPHIV_
toolkit/Documents/PresentationFiles/SlidesNotes_CLR.pdf. Used by permission
of FHI.

around puberty, so it is important to monitor whether this type of headache
suddenly starts during the teenage years.

Occasionally, the COCP can lead to an increase in blood pressure. Blood
pressure should be checked prior to commencing the COCP, and monitored
every 6 months until at least two consecutive stable normal BP readings
have been obtained. Annual BP monitoring should then be undertaken.

Educational support, perhaps from practice nurses about, for example, what
to do if a pill is missed, is very important for compliance. Teenage girls often
lead hectic lives, staying up late for homework deadlines or parties, catching up
on sleep at weekends, etc. Reminders, such as setting an alarm on a mobile
phone – a device that teenage girls are rarely seen without – can be very useful.

The combined pill works by suppressing the natural menstrual cycle, suppressing ovulation, and inducing a withdrawal bleed during the pill-free
week. Anovulatory cycles tend to be associated with lighter withdrawal
bleeds and less dysmenorrhoea, so these are further advantages to teenage
girls, offering them the potential to improve their heavy or painful periods.
If two packets of pills are taken consecutively, this avoids a withdrawal bleed
and can be useful for times when teenage girls want to skip a period (e.g. for
a holiday or swimming gala). This again enables them to have some control
over their periods at important times in their lives.

A new COCP is about to be launched in the UK, which will set the trend for other COCPs. These new regimes are based around 24 pills and four placebo tablets, instead of 21 pills and 7 pill-free days as previously. This new model of pill-taking offers advantages that will hopefully bring about a significant reduction of the current COCP failure rate. It is known that ovaries in about 10 per cent of COCP-takers show follicular activity by the seventh day of the pill-free break. This increases the potential for ovulation and consequent risk of pill-failure (i.e. pregnancy) if the first pill of the packet is missed or taken late. With the 24/4 regime, only 4 days are hormone-free (placebo days) and so:

1 ▷ the pill-taker does not have to remember to restart a pill regime after a break (which has been shown to increase pill-failure)
2 ▷ hormones are restarted after 4 hormone-free days rather than 7, so there is less likelihood of ovulation occurring.

The progesterone-only pill

The relatively new progesterone-only pill (POP) Cerazette appears to be a very safe pill, as it contains no oestrogen and so carries a negligible risk of DVT or stroke, and is safe to use in girls who suffer from migraine with aura. Cerazette is less popular than the COCP mainly because of the relatively common side effect of breakthrough bleeding.

About 1 in 3 girls will continue to have a monthly cycle on Cerazette. About 1 in 3 will have lighter bleeding (e.g. scantier or less frequent bleeds, or amenorrhoea), but about 1 in 3 will have nuisance spotting, more frequent bleeds or longer lasting bleeds. This group will understandably find Cerazette difficult to tolerate. They should be encouraged to persevere, however, as a number of them will settle into a more regular cycle after a few weeks. If Cerazette proves unacceptable and a COCP is contraindicated, they may need to try an alternative POP, which may or may not (it is really trial and error) settle down their bleeding pattern. The other POPs have the disadvantage of only providing 3 hours' leeway in which to remember to be taken. They work by thickening the cervical mucus, and this effect is lost relatively quickly if pills are missed or taken late. Cerazette has the additional benefit of suppressing ovulation in about 90 per cent of takers (unlike traditional POPs, which only suppress ovulation in about 30 per cent of takers), so for that 90 per cent Cerazette has the same 12 hours' leeway as the COCP. In teenage girls especially, acne can also be an undesirable side effect with POPs, including Cerazette, whereas some COCPs (e.g. Cilest and Yasmin) are 'skin-friendly' and actually improve acne.

Long-acting methods of contraception

Recent research has suggested that, in spite of some extra costs in the beginning, the reliability of these methods and the fact that they are not dependent on the memory and compliance of users means that these are actually more cost-effective than oral contraception. National Institute for Health and Clinical Excellence (NICE) guidelines recommend that the use of LARCs should be increased.[6]

IMPLANON

This is an implant of a progesterone molecule similar to Cerazette. It is fitted in the subcutaneous tissue of the arm under local anaesthetic and provides reliable contraception for 3 years. Unfortunately, it has a very similar side effect profile to Cerazette, including the risk of nuisance bleeding. It is therefore advisable to have a trial of Cerazette (usually for about 3 months) prior to Implanon fitting. This is so that the girl knows what sort of side effects she is likely to experience, and understands how much of a nuisance the erratic bleeding can be, before committing herself to 3 years of Implanon. Implanon is an expensive method if the device is removed after a short time, but is cost-effective if tolerated for the full 3 years, so counselling prior to fitting is very important and can reduce the number of early requests for removal.

CONTRACEPTIVE INJECTIONS

Depo-provera injections have traditionally been a popular contraceptive method with teenage girls, as they can be administered every 12 weeks, are very effective, and often induce amenorrhoea. In the short term, as with any progesterone-only method, depo can produce breakthrough bleeding, but perseverance with the method often allows this bleeding to settle and amenorrhoea commonly follows.

Recent research evidence has raised concerns about the long-term use of depo in young women, especially under the age of 25.[7] The dose of progesterone in depo is higher than that of any other progesterone-only contraceptive method. Not only does it thicken up cervical mucus, but it also commonly suppresses ovulation. There is concern that it may even reduce oestrogen secretion by the ovaries, and this has implications for the long-term risk of osteoporosis. Bone is continually being broken down and rebuilt, but the rebuilding function is dependent on an adequate level of oestrogen. Furthermore, maximum bone density is usually not achieved in women until the age of about 24, so teenage girls using depo as a long-term method (say for 3 years, but possibly even less) risk not achieving their bone density potential if low oestrogen levels interfere with their osteoblastic bone-building activity.

To keep the above concerns in perspective, the research mentioned[7] has been criticised because the group using depo-provera has been shown to contain a higher proportion of smokers (another risk factor for lowering bone density) whilst the comparison group contains women on the COCP (which contains oestrogen, which is of benefit to bone rebuilding). Depo-provera is however the only contraceptive method that has been linked with any possible risk of osteoporosis so informed consent should be ensured and alternatives should usually be discussed.

INTRAUTERINE CONTRACEPTIVE DEVICE

The copper coil, or intrauterine contraceptive device (IUCD), is not a particular favourite with teenage girls, but does definitely have a place, as it is an extremely cost-effective LARC. However, certain potential side effects must be considered and explained for an informed choice to be made:

1 ▷ Statistically, there is a small but significant rise in reported pelvic infections in the first 3 weeks after an IUCD fitting. This may be mainly due to previously asymptomatic infections in the cervix (e.g. chlamydia) being spread further up the genital tract at the time of fitting, and can lead to infertility. The incidence of these infections can be reduced by screening and treating prior to IUCD fitting. If screening results cannot be made available in time, e.g. in a postcoital IUCD fitting, then antibiotic cover should be given.

2 ▷ There is a risk of ectopic pregnancy. The copper IUCD works mainly by killing sperm, but if an ovum is fertilised the high copper levels in the uterus normally prevent implantation and the egg disintegrates. Because there are lower levels of copper from the IUCD in the fallopian tubes, attempts at implantation here are more likely to be successful than in the uterus. This means that a higher proportion of pregnancies conceived with an IUCD *in situ* are ectopic pregnancies than in pregnancies occurring with other forms of contraception, although the IUCD does not increase the risk of an ectopic pregnancy as compared with unprotected sex.

MIRENA INTRAUTERINE SYSTEM

This is not a commonly used contraceptive method in teenage girls. It has a slightly wider-fitting tube than the IUCD so is technically a little more difficult, but can be aided by the use of local anaesthetic in the form of a cervical block. Like all progesterone-only methods, it can cause erratic bleeding in the first few months of use. However, it can be very helpful for long-term use in menorrhagia and dysmenorrhoea, and it is a very effective contraceptive method. The same infection screening prior to fitting should be undertaken as with an IUCD, to prevent the spread of pelvic infection.

Other methods of contraception

There are some relatively new methods of contraception, but these do not seem to be as popular in the UK as they are in the USA. The Ortho Evra patch and the NuvaRing are both alternative methods of delivering combined oestrogen and progesterone contraception. They are considerably more expensive than the COCP, but probably carry the same clinical risks. The patch needs to be applied once a week for 3 weeks, followed by a week without a patch. The manufacturers provide a weekly text to a mobile phone to remind users who register with them that they need to apply their patch. Recent evidence suggests that serum oestradiol levels are considerably higher with the patch than with the COCP, and this raises concerns about DVT risk.[8] This has led to the US Food and Drug Administration updating the Ortho Evra contraceptive patch labelling to warn that the patch exposes users to 60 per cent more total oestrogen than typical COCPs.[9]

The NuvaRing is a vaginal ring, worn for 3 weeks and removed for 1 week. It delivers combined contraception, but is not really a popular choice with teenage girls, because they do not always feel confident or comfortable fitting something inside their vagina. Research suggests that the oestradiol levels from the NuvaRing may be significantly lower than with the COCP, so there is a possibility that this might be a safer method of administration with a view to DVT risk, but further research would need to be done to investigate this.[8]

Condoms

Ideally, condoms should not be used as the sole method of contraception, but always be used as well as another contraceptive method, i.e. the 'double Dutch' method, named for its common use in the Netherlands. Although condoms alone are not a particularly reliable form of contraception in practice, they do help reduce transmission of sexually transmitted infections (STIs), and their use should, therefore, be encouraged at every opportunity. Their reliability for both contraception and STI prevention is dependent on the way they are used, so teenagers especially need to have explicit instruction on how to use condoms.

Emergency contraception

Teenage girls may not be very good at pre-planning, and so may often need emergency contraception. If they attend within 72 hours of unprotected sex, they can be treated with Levonelle 1500. They should also be advised that the emergency copper IUCD fitting is the most dependable method of emergency contraception between 72 hours and 120 hours post-exposure. If declined, then Levonelle 1500 should still be considered. Although it is only licensed to be prescribed up to 72 hours postcoitally, it is still effective (although considerably less so) beyond this time window. It has been shown to be safe even if pregnancy is not prevented, with no evidence of teratogenicity.

Sexually transmitted infections

Teenagers are at particular risk of STIs, as they tend to have shorter-lived relationships than adults and to change their partners more often. They also may be prone to risk-taking behaviour, and so more at risk of the consequences of unsafe sex, such as unplanned pregnancy and STIs, including HIV infection.

The incidence of STIs in the UK, especially chlamydia but including gonorrhoea and genital herpes, has been steadily rising. Fortunately, rates in the under-16s have remained relatively low, but in older teenagers the incidence has increased dramatically.[1] Symptoms are similar to those in adults, although chlamydia (which is often asymptomatic in women) is more likely to present with vaginal discharge in teenage girls. However, in the majority of cases it is completely asymptomatic, and so screening should always be considered. Breakthrough bleeding on any form of contraception, from the pill to the IUCD to the implant, should be considered as a possible marker for an STI and this really needs to be ruled out prior to further investigations.

Unfortunately, the immature cervix of teenage girls appears to make them more susceptible to chlamydia infection. Chlamydia has important long-term consequences if untreated, including pelvic infection, ectopic pregnancy and infertility. There is a national chlamydia screening programme now in place, which invites girls and women under the age of 25 to be screened opportunistically in primary care for chlamydia with a self-sampled low-vaginal swab or urine sample. This has the advantage of being used with new highly sensitive nucleic acid amplification tests. However, progress towards eradication of chlamydia in the teenage population depends on compliance and concordance with treatment, and on successful partner treatment, which will not always be straightforward as relation-ships may be brief, and partner details may not be easy to obtain.

Immunisations

A recent major change to the immunisation schedule for adolescents is the start of the human papillomavirus or wart virus (HPV) immunisation programme for girls aged 12–13 years.[10] The vaccine protects against HPV types 16 and 18, which are associated with increased risk of cervical cancer. Through the changes they induce in the nucleus of the cells of the cervix, they are thought to be the cause of about 70 per cent of cases of cervical cancer.[11]

Two vaccines are available, Gardasil and Cervarix. The UK government has chosen Cervarix as the vaccine to be used in the national immunisation programme. Both protect against HPV 16 and HPV 18, but Gardasil also protects against HPV 6 and HPV 11, which cause about 90 per cent of genital wart cases. Cervarix alone protects against the less common types HPV 31 and HPV 45. There is speculation that the choice of Cervarix in the UK was mainly determined by cost issues, and Gardasil is being used in the USA to vaccinate both boys and girls. However, the *New York Post* revealed on 6 July 2008 that Gardasil is under investigation for possible links to paralysis, seizures and 18 deaths.[12] Gardasil is currently available privately in the UK, as an alternative to Cervarix.

The introduction of the Cervarix immunisation programme has been sur-rounded by controversy. Not only are parents wary of the potential side effects of a new vaccine, but some parents, and schools (where the vaccine is to be administered nationwide), have also expressed fears of encouraging promiscuous behaviour in girls by vaccinating them at such a young age. However, there is no evidence that prophylaxis against STIs encourages promiscuous behaviour.

Further, any girl may still be at risk of acquiring HPV and consequently cervical cancer. The incidence of 'teen date violence', which often involves rape or sexual assault of a teenage girl by a boy or man she is dating, con-tinues to increase. US figures show that approximately 1 in 10 high school students experiences sexual dating violence – that figure is 22 per cent in college students.[13]

One further aspect that remains to be resolved is that of consent where a girl may wish to be immunised, but her parents are against it, or vice versa.

Teenage pregnancy

The incidence of unplanned teenage pregnancy varies widely between countries, and the UK tops most countries in Europe. Through the 1970s, 1980s and 1990s, teenage birth rates fell in most of Western Europe, but have remained high in the UK, in spite of government targets to reduce them.

There are some groups of women, e.g. some South Asian ethnic groups, where teenage pregnancy rates are high among young married women and are a positive choice. However, many are unplanned and have major implications for the lives and future plans of the teenage mothers.

Figure 13.2 shows the variation in live birth rates around the world in teenagers.[14]

Figure 13.2 ○ *Birth rates among teenagers aged 15–19 in 1998*

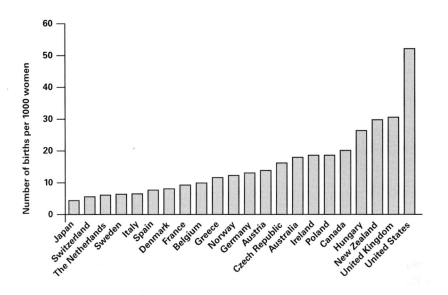

Source: UNICEF, 'A league table of teenage births in rich nations', *Innocenti Report Card* No.3, July 2001. UNICEF Innocenti Research Centre, Florence.

The strongest risk factor for teenage pregnancy is poverty. There is also evidence that social exclusion may increase teenage pregnancy risk. Social exclusion entails 'individuals being disadvantaged not just economically but also in terms of other dimensions such as education, citizenship and cultural resources.'[15] For teenagers, this often means a lack of interest and 'belonging' in school and school-related activities. Factors that protect against teenage pregnancy include high interest in school activity, strong family support, strong religious beliefs, and a stable relationship with a partner.[1]

Teenage pregnancy rates in Canada and the USA have been significantly higher than in Europe but there has been a reduction over the past 15 years. Between 1994 and 2002, pregnancy rates per 1000 girls aged 15–19 increased from 58.7 to 60.3 in England and Wales, whereas they fell from 106.1 to 76.4 in the USA. Studies have shown that this fall was due to increased use of contraception among teenagers.[16] Canadian statistics showed a fall similar to the USA trend (from 49.2 to 33.9).[16] Interestingly, abortion rates in this age group are higher in England and Wales than in the USA, with abortions standing at 24.1 per 1000 girls aged 15–19 in England and Wales compared with 21.7 in the USA.[16]

Summary

▷ Contraception and sexual health care can be provided to a teenage girl without the consent of an adult, as long as she is deemed to be competent to consent to treatment and as long as the relationship seems to be completely her choice, without any external influences.

▷ STIs are common in sexually active teenagers and always need to be considered. One of the commonest ways they can present (especially chlamydia) is as 'breakthrough bleeding' with any contraceptive method. Any teenage girl presenting with breakthrough bleeding should be assessed for STI risk and probably screened. This involves good communication skills on the part of the health practitioner and taking a clear, specific and non-judgemental sexual history.

▷ There is a relatively new national screening and treatment programme for chlamydia in young women and girls. However, the success of this depends on opportunistic screening and treatment of contacts.

▷ There is a new immunisation programme nationally for the two HPV types most commonly associated with cervical cancer.

▷ Unplanned teenage pregnancies are high in the UK, one of the highest rates in Europe.

▷ LARCs have been shown to be more cost-effective than oral contraception and increased usage should be encouraged in teenagers, as recommended by NICE.

193

How does the GP curriculum help us think about the care of this group of patients?

Primary care management

▷ Teenagers have special needs in primary care, including a requirement for ease of access outside school hours and confidentiality.

Person-centred care

▷ Talking to teenagers requires all our expertise and communication skills. Teenagers can be seen alone, but only if they appear to have the capacity to understand and make informed decisions, as judged by the Fraser guidelines.[3]

Specific problem-solving skills

▷ The requirements to protect teenagers from unplanned pregnancy as well as infections may not always be easy to meet, but options are available and need to be tailored to each individual patient.

A comprehensive approach

▷ A low threshold for screening for STIs is necessary, as teenagers are at high risk and they are asymptomatic in the majority of cases. Contact tracing is very important.

Community orientation

▷ The place of a teenager in society is different from that of an independent adult. Their bodies may still be growing and changing through puberty. They often have ongoing educational needs. They may also be subject to cultural influences. They are old enough to want to be independent, but still vulnerable enough to need the protection of society.

A holistic approach

▷ Any suspicion of a child protection issue must take priority over issues of confidentiality and capacity. Even if a teenage girl appears to have the capacity to understand what she is doing, and appears to be consenting to what is happening, she may still be vulnerable to peer pressure and pressures of adults in a position of power over her. The healthcare professional she confides in needs always to consider whether she is being unduly influenced against free choice.

Case discussion

Consider the case of Kerry, aged 15.

▶ Kerry is a 15-year-old girl who consults you, saying that she has been having a sexual relationship with her 16-year-old boyfriend for the past 3 weeks. They have just fallen out because she found out that he had had sex with two other girls in her class before her. She feels 'used' and she is also worried about the possibility of pregnancy.

▷ What are the main areas to be considered and what would be your first steps?

It has possibly taken a lot for Kerry to be able to make an appointment and come to see you. Has she come alone? She might have had to miss school and lied to her parents to make an appointment. Does she feel unsupported? You will need a non-judgemental supportive style to build a rapport.

RISK OF PREGNANCY

▶ Levonelle 1500 within 72 hours could protect her for the most recent sexual encounter but not for previous encounters that cycle. If she is within 5 days of unprotected sexual intercourse, she could be suitable for an emergency IUCD fitting. In this case, if she was not using contraception, it is too late to be able to do anything to prevent pregnancy, but we can prepare her for the possibility and ensure that a pregnancy test is arranged.

Risk of STI

▶ This could certainly be a possibility if her ex-boyfriend's reported sexual history is true, and she would need counselling and information leaflets about this possibility, plus screening for STIs. She should be screened on her first visit to you in case the courage it has taken to attend fails her and she does not return.

Kerry may be quite emotionally disturbed about these events. She may feel 'used' and 'dirty'. She may feel silly for thinking that she meant something more to her boyfriend, and her self-esteem may have taken a heavy blow. She may also feel angry with the other girls concerned, and that she cannot trust girls that she thought were her friends. It is not uncommon for teenage girls to self-harm or even make serious attempts at suicide in these emotional situations. Kerry may need some emotional support/counselling over the next few weeks. A good start to a relationship with you at this stage will be important.

References

1 • Tripp J, Viner R. ABC of adolescence: sexual health, contraception, and teenage pregnancy *British Medical Journal* 2005; **330**: 590–3.

2 • McPherson A. Adolescents in primary care *British Medical Journal* 2005; **330**: 465–7.

3 • www.confidentiality.scot.nhs.uk/fraser_guidelines.htm [accessed August 2009].

4 • Larcher V. ABC of adolescence: consent, competence and confidentiality *British Medical Journal* 2005; **330**: 353–6.

5 • Trussell, 1994; Jones/Forrest, 1992 (COC typical use data).

6 • National Collaborating Centre for Women's and Children's Health. *Long-Acting Reversible Contraception: the effective and appropriate use of long-acting reversible contraception* London: RCOG Press, 2005.

7 • Medicines and Healthcare products Regulatory Agency. www.mhra.gov.uk [accessed August 2009].

8 • van den Heuvel M W, van Bragt A J, Alnabawy A K, *et al*. Comparison of ethinylestradiol pharmacokinetics in three hormonal contraceptive formulations: the vaginal ring, the transdermal patch and an oral contraceptive *Contraception* 2005; **72**: 168–74.

9 • US Food and Drug Administration. *A Public Health Advisory: Ortho Evra* Silver Spring, MD: FDA, 2005.

10 • Department of Health. *Immunisation against Infectious Disease* ['The Green Book'] Norwich: TSO, 2006.

11 • NHS Direct. *HPV Vaccination* http://cks.library.nhs.uk/patient_information_leaflet/hpv_vaccination [accessed August 2009].

12 • *New York Post*, 6 July 2008.

13 • Wilson K J. *When Violence Begins at Home: a comprehensive guide to understanding and ending domestic abuse* California: Hunter House Inc. Publishers, 1997.

14 • Brennan K. Increasing incidence of sexually transmitted infections in UK [news] *Student BMJ* 2002; **10(95)**: 215–58.

15 • Bonnell C P, Strange V J, Stephenson J M, *et al*. 'Effect of social exclusion' on the risk of teenage pregnancy: development of hypotheses using baseline data from a randomized trial of sex education *Journal of Epidemiology and Community Health* 2003: **57**: 871–6.

16 • Langille D B. Teenage pregnancy: trends, contributing factors and the physician's role *Canadian Medical Association Journal* 2007; **176(11)**: 1601–2.

Substance misuse and addiction in adolescence

Issues for the practising GP

Ilana Crome

Introduction

Young people in the UK have some of the highest rates of substance misuse in Europe.[1] They are highly likely to present to primary care with substance-related problems.

Substance misuse is a substantial public health issue with considerable mortality and morbidity. Depression and anxiety, self-harm and suicide, cirrhosis, and criminality, as well as many other psychological, physical, and social harms can result.

The age at which young people start using substances and experiencing problems is getting earlier and the historical gap between higher use in boys compared with girls is narrowing. For some substances at some ages girls are using more than boys.

It is important that GPs feel confident about undertaking an assessment that places the substance use in the context of the young person's life. The primary healthcare team has a central role in recognition, treatment and collaborating with specialist health and social services to provide the young person and his or her family and carers with the appropriate level of support. Treatment can be successful, especially if difficulties are spotted early and a comprehensive, cohesive child-centred approach is organised.

Some facts[2-6]

▷ Drug problems are estimated to cost the country about £15 billion per annum.
▷ Alcohol problems are estimated to cost the country about £20 billion per annum.
▷ There are approximately 120,000 premature deaths from cigarette smoking each year.

▷ There are about 22,000 premature deaths from alcohol misuse each year.
▷ There are 2000–3000 deaths from drug misuse each year.
▷ The overall mortality of adolescent addicts is 16 times that of the general adolescent population.

Young people constitute about one-sixth of the population (or 6.8 million in England and Wales).
In 15-year-olds:[3]

▷ 20–25 per cent are regular smokers
▷ 40–50 per cent drink alcohol weekly
▷ 20–25 per cent use other drugs (mainly cannabis) at least monthly.

In the 16–24-year-old age group:[7]

▷ 1.5 million used one or more illicit drugs in the past year
▷ 1.3 million used cannabis in the past year
▷ over 530,000 used a Class A drug in the past year
▷ 2.1 million are daily smokers
▷ 1.9 million exceed the recommended adult safe limits for alcohol at least once a month.

This chapter aims to cover the following key learning points:

▷ the extent of and difference between substance use, misuse and dependence
▷ the factors that predispose to substance use, those that might mitigate the effects of use, and those that are protective
▷ how to undertake a comprehensive assessment that places the substance use in the context of the young person's development, family, educational attainment, social network and community values
▷ the range of pharmacological treatments that are available for young people and when prescribing is appropriate
▷ the range of psychological interventions that may be beneficial and those that are suitable for primary care settings
▷ the role of the primary care team in assessment, treatment and liaison with specialist health services and social care
▷ the legal and ethical issues with regard to confidentiality and consent.

Prevalence: the scale of the problem

Cigarettes and alcohol are the most commonly abused substances.[3,8] Box 14.1 lists some key facts.

Box 14.1 ○ *Prevalence of drug misuse*

Alcohol

▷ Alcohol consumption has doubled over the last 50 years.[9]

▷ Young drinkers aged 11–15 in England doubled their average weekly consumption from 5.3 units in 1990 to 10.2 in 2002.[9] Since this time, consumption has stabilised in boys but continues to increase in girls.

▷ The proportion of children who drink increases with age.

▷ Twenty-one per cent of children aged 11–15 drank alcohol in the previous week.[6]

▷ Forty-five per cent of young people aged 16–24 exceeded the daily benchmark of two units for females and three for males.

▷ Among young women aged 16–24 the percentage exceeding the daily benchmark has more than doubled from 15 per cent in 1988–9 to 33 per cent in 2002–3. Forty per cent exceeded three units on at least one day in the previous week.[10,11]

Cigarettes

▷ The prevalence of cigarette smoking is higher among 20–24-year-olds than in any other age group, despite a fall in overall prevalence.[12]

▷ In 2004, 7 per cent of boys aged 11–15 in England were regular smokers (that is, they usually smoked at least one cigarette a week), compared with 10 per cent of girls.

Illicit drugs

▷ One and a half million young people aged 16–24 have used an illicit drug over the past year.[13] Men more commonly report use.

▷ In 2005, one in ten secondary school children in England reported using drugs in the month prior to interview, while one in five reported using drugs in the year prior to interview.

▷ Thirty-three per cent of young men aged 16–24 reported use of any illicit drug in the past year in 2004–5, but for their female counterparts it was 21 per cent.[14]

▷ Twenty-six per cent of young adults aged 16–24 reported using drugs in the year prior to interview in England and Wales in 2004–5. Sixteen per cent had used drugs in the month prior to interview. Almost half (45.8 per cent) reported that they had ever used drugs.

Harms associated with substance misuse

GPs are well placed to recognise the physical and mental health problems with which young people might present.[15] There is increasing appreciation that mental disorders that start in childhood may continue into adult life, especially if they are not recognised and treated early. The risks to health might be a result of the acute impact of the substance or substances, but can also result from associated behaviours such as sexual activity and dependency needs. These young people may take a combination of substances, may genuinely not know what they have taken, and may swallow, inhale, smoke and inject substances. They may have minimal knowledge of the risks involved.

The risks include:

▷ intoxication, leading to coma, vomiting, hypothermia, injury and accidents
▷ withdrawal syndrome – each drug has a particular set of withdrawal symptoms, some of which may be life threatening, e.g. delirium tremens from alcohol withdrawal, or depression, inertia and even suicide from stimulant withdrawal (see Table 14.1, pp. 202–3)
▷ smoking and inhalation, which may lead to a persistent cough, exacerbation of asthma or perforation of nasal septum (cocaine), and cancer
▷ overdose, suicide and self-harm, which may be accidental or deliberate and may result from combinations of drugs or the effects of individual drugs, e.g. stimulants may lead to cardiac arrest
▷ infections that may have been caused by injecting, e.g. HIV, hepatitis B and C, septicaemia, thrombophlebitis, abscesses, ulcers and deep vein thrombosis
▷ chronic substance misuse, which may have generalised effects of poor nutrition, unpredictability, agitation and irritability, as well as specific acute and chronic effects
▷ young people becoming victims of exploitation and abuse, and becoming involved in prostitution – sexual behaviour and substance use are interrelated in many complex ways
▷ poor diet and eating disorders, which are linked for example to laxatives and opiate use and stimulant use for weight loss
▷ affective disorders, e.g. depression, anxiety, panic, phobia
▷ post-traumatic stress syndrome
▷ attention deficit hyperactivity syndrome
▷ psychotic illness, which is associated with the use of stimulants and cannabis
▷ personality problems, including conduct, borderline and antisocial personality disorders.

Risk and protective factors

Some of the risk factors for substance misuse include genetic predisposition, prenatal exposure to drugs, psychopathology, e.g. conduct disorder and antisocial behaviour, depression, and attention deficit hyperactivity disorder (ADHD). In the home environment and parenting the risk factors are, for example, physical, sexual and emotional abuse; neglect, lack of warmth, lack of supervision; aggression, hostility and domestic violence.

Protective factors can act at the individual, family and community levels, and their interaction is complex. Individual protective factors include high intelligence, positive self-esteem, personal and social competence, and a sense of independence or autonomy. Familial protective factors include strong parental attachment, someone in whom to confide and family cohesion. Clearly defined social norms about substance use can be protective.

Young people who fall into the following groups appear to be at a high risk of developing a substance misuse problem. These include those:

▷ whose parents misuse substances
▷ whose parents have a psychiatric illness
▷ from dysfunctional families
▷ with mental health problems
▷ with a history of self-harm
▷ who frequently attend accident and emergency services
▷ with a history of abuse.

And also:

▷ pregnant teenage women
▷ looked-after young people
▷ homeless young people
▷ young offenders
▷ young people who do not attend school regularly
▷ young people with chaotic lifestyles.

201

Diagnosing dependence (addiction)

The term 'substance use' applies to legal use that is acceptable socially and without impairment of social, psychological or physical functioning. Misuse should be applied to use that is unlawful or which is not socially or medically approved, and which has the potential to cause harm. Harmful use, according to ICD-10 classification, is where 'substance use contributed to physical or psychological harm'.[16]

Substance use may be suspected from the behaviours, symptoms and signs listed in Table 14.1 (pp. 202–3).

Table 14.1 ○ **Symptoms of intoxication and withdrawal**[15]

Substance	Intoxication	Withdrawal
Alcohol	Disinhibition	Tremor (tongue, eyelids, hands)
	Argumentativeness	Agitation, insomnia, malaise
	Aggression	Convulsions
	Interference with personal functioning	Visual, auditory, tactile illusions or hallucinations
	Labile mood	
	Impaired judgement and attention	
	Unsteady gait and difficulty in standing	
	Slurred speech	
	Nystagmus	
	Decreased level of consciousness	
	Flushed face	
	Conjunctival injection	
Opiates	Apathy	Craving
	Sedation, drowsiness, slurred speech	Sneezing, yawning, runny eyes
	Disinhibition	Muscle aches, abdominal pains
	Psychomotor retardation	Nausea, vomiting, diarrhoea
	Impaired attention and judgement	Goose flesh, recurrent chills
	Pupillary constriction	Pupillary dilatation
	Decreased level of consciousness	Restless sleep
	Interference with personal functioning	
Cannabis	Euphoria and disinhibition	Anxiety
	Anxiety and agitation	Irritability
	Suspiciousness and paranoid ideation	Tremor
	Impaired reaction time, judgement and attention	Sweating
	Hallucinations with preserved orientation	Muscle aches

Substance	Intoxication	Withdrawal
Cannabis	Depersonalisation and derealisation	
	Increased appetite	
	Dry mouth	
	Conjunctival injection	
	Tachycardia	
Nicotine	Insomnia	Craving
	Bizarre dreams	Malaise or weakness
	Fluctuating mood	Anxiety, irritability, moodiness
	Derealisation	Insomnia
	Interference with personal functioning	Increased appetite
	Nausea	Increased cough and mouth ulceration
	Sweating	Difficulty concentrating
		Tachycardia and cardiac arrhythmias
Stimulants	Euphoria and increased energy	Lethargy
	Hypervigilance	Psychomotor retardation or agitation
	Repetitive stereotyped behaviours	Craving
	Grandiose beliefs and actions	Increased appetite
	Paranoid ideation	Insomnia or hypersomnia
	Abusiveness, aggression and argumentativeness	Bizarre and unpleasant dreams
	Auditory, tactile and visual hallucinations	
	Sweats, chills, muscular weakness	
	Nausea or vomiting, weight loss	
	Pupillary dilatation, convulsions	
	Tachycardia, arrhythmias, chest pain, hypertension	
	Agitation	

Although only a minority of young people develop dependence, it is imperative that you are able to distinguish between substance use, misuse and dependence because this has a bearing on the type of treatment modalities that you might consider. For example, pharmacological agents are used when patients are dependent for the purposes of detoxification or substitution.

A diagnosis of dependence can be made if three of the following criteria have been present during the preceding 12 months:

▷ compulsion or craving, i.e. a strong desire to take the substance
▷ tolerance, i.e. needing more to get the same effect
▷ difficulties in controlling the use of substances
▷ a withdrawal syndrome when substance use is reduced or stopped
▷ relief of withdrawal by substance use
▷ persistent use despite evidence of harmful consequences
▷ neglect of interests and an increased amount of time taken to obtain the substance or to recover from its effects.

Consider the case histories in Box 14.2 and the treatment approaches that can be used in each case. Good care is not just a matter of prescribing (which must be undertaken by trained, experienced staff in the context of many other medical and social problems) but needs the full range of professionals to work together. Facilities required include supported accommodation, general medical and dental practitioners, child and adolescent psychiatric support, family therapy and crisis intervention. Think about the dilemmas of disengagement in this exceedingly vulnerable group and the transitional aspects of care.

Box 14.2 ○ *Case histories*

Jake is 15 years' old and is injecting heroin. He is an only child, not in school, and is under-weight, having lost several stones in a few months. His physical appearance is poor. He is escorted by his mother, with her boyfriend.
His mother seems genuinely concerned and close to her son, but is very suspicious of services and involvement of others. The boy is articulate and able to seek support.

Emma, 16, who has recently registered at your practice presents to you complaining of anxiety and sleeping difficulties. She visits you a few times and does not appear to be improving, although she is very pleasant and placid. You discover that she is living with a new partner who you know is a drug user and who is 10 years older than she is. She is living away from her family. Eventually, she reluctantly admits that she is using small amounts of heroin and may be pregnant.

Katie, 13 years' old, is referred to you from school due to alcohol use affecting her school attendance and work. She has been falling asleep in lessons, has been disruptive and has not attended regularly.

With Jake, you need to gain trust in order to undertake an initial assessment. What would your immediate concerns and the immediate risks be? His mother is not a patient at your surgery, though his grandfather is. Would you enquire further about his mother's background?

You decide to carry out some blood tests and do a physical check-up. You will need to be flexible about attendance, as vulnerable young people are often late for appointments or may even miss them without cancelling.

It soon starts to become apparent that Jake's physical appearance is worsening. He is accessing needles through others and is not being supported to attend doctor's and other appointments. You could recommend the local needle exchange and may decide that this young person should be referred to the local adolescent addiction service. There is so much concern that on one occasion the drugs worker actively escorts him, with his mother, from the GP's surgery to attend the young person's service. His mother is still hostile towards the service and in particular the drugs worker, and questions the confidentiality policy. How much effort would you place on supporting this mother, independently of the young man? If the family disengaged, what would you do?

Let us consider Emma. Her pregnancy goes well but the baby is blind and has endocrine problems. She has been attending the adolescent addiction service for 18 months and is relatively stable on methadone. She attends reliably and uses support for her baby well. However, her life is stressful given her child's difficulties. As her partner uses, she is tempted to 'use on top', adding illicit drugs on top of her prescription, and is on the verge of feeling that she may need an increased dose of methadone. She has never had a negative urine screen. Think about how you could handle this situation, and in particular which other agencies you will need to bring to support Emma and the baby.

Katie is very young and vulnerable. Where would you consider the most appropriate setting to assess her? What would be the key elements of the assessment that you would consider important for planning treatment further? Your view is that the alcohol use is affecting all aspects of her life. How would you relate this to her parents, with whom she is living? What help would you offer Katie and her parents or family? How would you ensure that her education is not further disrupted and that she is not excluded from school?

Primary care management

A vital component of primary care involvement is a comprehensive assessment and history taking. This may take place over several occasions, as situations may change very rapidly in the lives of young people. You will need to ask questions about route of use, quantity, frequency of use, combinations of substances, pattern of use, and associated problems.

The impact of this use on the young person's physical, psychological and social wellbeing needs to be ascertained, to what extent the safety of the young person is compromised, and whether there is a need for therapeutic intervention. It is important to intervene with young people as early as possible because use at a very early age is recognised as a predictor of later substance misuse and dependence. The maturity of the young person must also be assessed, as this affects consent and, more importantly, refusal of treatment (see Chapter 12). Although motivation for psychological change is difficult to assess, some attempt should be made to determine what had led to the presentation in primary care, so that this first contact maximises engagement. It is important that harm reduction is considered, as well as cessation. Advice should be accurate, credible and appropriate to the young person.

Treatment options

Over the last two decades there has been accumulating evidence that treatment for substance problems in adults can be effective.[15, 17, 18] As young people have different needs, these findings cannot be directly applied to young people. It is still possible to treat young people safely and effectively by systematically and cautiously implementing treatments tried and tested in the adult population in settings and with safeguards that are appropriate for young people. It is not generally appropriate to treat young people in adult facilities.

Evidence for the treatment of young substance misusers is sparse, especially in terms of UK-based studies.[19-22] Published guidelines on substance misuse from the National Institute of Health and Clinical Excellence (NICE) are not always relevant to young people and the evidence on which they are based may not include patients within this age range.[23-26]

Research into outcomes of young people treated in substance misuse services in the USA demonstrate that they can be very variable, but that up to about 50 per cent of patients do improve and achieve abstinence or a reduction in substance use several years after treatment.[27, 28] Encouragingly, some decrease from pre-treatment levels of use is demonstrated in most studies.[29, 30] Dropout rates however are high and patients are likely to have co-morbid conditions. Improvements in problem behaviour, criminal activity, mental health, school attendance and family relationships following treatment have been reported, mainly in the USA.[20, 31-33]

Care in the primary care team

Provision of information and advice for young people and their families

Posters, leaflets and brochures can be scattered around the surgery with contact details for addiction support services locally. Every consultation is an opportunity to consider the role of substances in the presentation.

Psychological treatments

Brief intervention, motivational interviewing, cognitive behavioural therapy (CBT), family therapies, and support and community reinforcement generally demonstrate promising results in substance use and other behaviours over 12 months' follow-up.[20–22, 34–36]

Pharmacological treatment

Most pharmacological agents are not licensed for adolescents and initiation of pharmacological treatment should generally only be offered by specialist addiction psychiatrists or similarly experienced and qualified practitioners in primary care. Young people may also need medication for psychiatric illness and physical problems, some of which may interact with each other. Risks of overdose must be explained to the patient, family and carers, and contact details of appropriate services provided to them. Table 14.2 (p. 208) lists current recommended drug treatments that may be useful. If drugs are not licensed for use in young people, it does not mean that they cannot be used. However, it implies that special care needs to be taken if prescribing does take place.

Specialist service provision for adolescent substance misusers is geographically patchy and the components of service models are very variable.[37] Services are often based on the interests and entrepreneurship of the teams; the resources to implement evidence-based treatment or to evaluate and test novel approaches are inadequate. In order to find out what resources are available in your area, information can be obtained from the National Treatment Agency's website and regional offices (see www.nta.nhs.uk/).[38]

Although substance use and misuse is very common in young people, and is often a one-off phenomenon, it is occasionally fatal and should be taken seriously. It is not necessarily 'a phase' a young person is going through. If identified early, there is the opportunity to treat associated psychosocial and physical problems, and to prevent deterioration. Even if the young person presents with a range of problems, there is benefit in reduction or abstinence, i.e. a downward spiral is not inevitable.

Table 14.2 ○ *Licensing of pharmacological treatments for use in young people with substance misuse*

Medication	Licensed	Age limits	Specific recommendations
Diazepam	Alcohol withdrawal	Not in children	< half adult dose in anxiety
Chlordiazepoxide	Alcohol withdrawal	Not in children	< half adult dose in anxiety
Disulfiram	Alcohol deterrent	Not in children	None
Methadone	Opiate addiction	Not in children	Caution
Subutex	Opiate addiction	> 16 years	None
Lofexidine	Opiate detoxification	Not in children	Caution
Nicotine replacement therapy	Nicotine withdrawal	> 18 years	None
Bupropion	Smoking cessation	> 18 years	Caution

Source: adapted from *British National Formulary* 2009: **57**.

There is a number of NHS and voluntary organisations that provide support. Onward referral and liaison with specialist services may be necessary for the following:

▷ misuse of multiple substances
▷ severe dependence
▷ frequent relapses of substance misuse
▷ co-morbid severe physical illness
▷ co-morbid severe mental illness
▷ unstable accommodation, including homelessness
▷ family disharmony or dysfunction
▷ chaotic lifestyle, with little structure or support.

Clinical governance issues

Confidentiality and access to services specifically designed for young people need specific consideration. Primary care teams and other local services should have well-formulated policies on confidentiality and consent for young people and their families. If GPs are taking a central role in the management of substance misuse, especially prescribing, then there should be a clear management structure and an accountability framework within which they are operating to protect the patient, the practitioner and the practice.[39]

Supervision and discussion about cases should be undertaken on a regular basis. Young substance misusers may have a very high level of risk with a degree of unpredictability.

However, to conclude, they are a joy to work with and the work can be extremely rewarding.

Appendix: assessment flow charts

Figure 14.1 ○ *A framework for assessment*

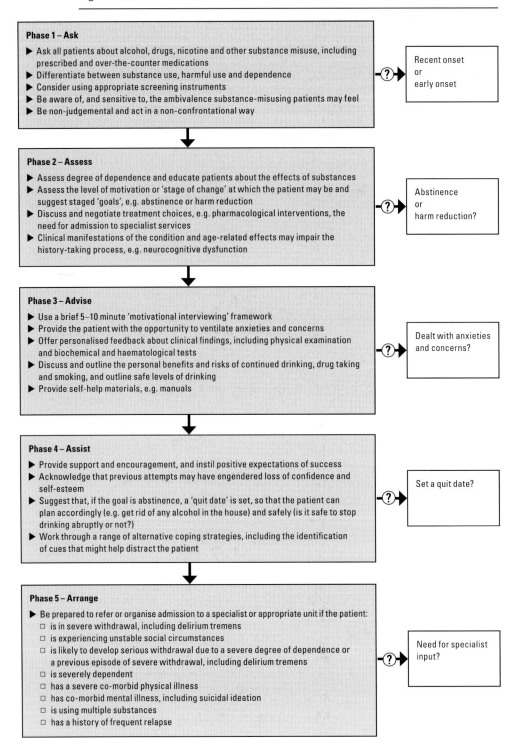

Phase 1 – Ask

▶ Ask all patients about alcohol, drugs, nicotine and other substance misuse, including prescribed and over-the-counter medications
▶ Differentiate between substance use, harmful use and dependence
▶ Consider using appropriate screening instruments
▶ Be aware of, and sensitive to, the ambivalence substance-misusing patients may feel
▶ Be non-judgemental and act in a non-confrontational way

⟶ ⟨?⟩ ⟶ Recent onset or early onset

Phase 2 – Assess

▶ Assess degree of dependence and educate patients about the effects of substances
▶ Assess the level of motivation or 'stage of change' at which the patient may be and suggest staged 'goals', e.g. abstinence or harm reduction
▶ Discuss and negotiate treatment choices, e.g. pharmacological interventions, the need for admission to specialist services
▶ Clinical manifestations of the condition and age-related effects may impair the history-taking process, e.g. neurocognitive dysfunction

⟶ ⟨?⟩ ⟶ Abstinence or harm reduction?

Phase 3 – Advise

▶ Use a brief 5–10 minute 'motivational interviewing' framework
▶ Provide the patient with the opportunity to ventilate anxieties and concerns
▶ Offer personalised feedback about clinical findings, including physical examination and biochemical and haematological tests
▶ Discuss and outline the personal benefits and risks of continued drinking, drug taking and smoking, and outline safe levels of drinking
▶ Provide self-help materials, e.g. manuals

⟶ ⟨?⟩ ⟶ Dealt with anxieties and concerns?

Phase 4 – Assist

▶ Provide support and encouragement, and instil positive expectations of success
▶ Acknowledge that previous attempts may have engendered loss of confidence and self-esteem
▶ Suggest that, if the goal is abstinence, a 'quit date' is set, so that the patient can plan accordingly (e.g. get rid of any alcohol in the house) and safely (is it safe to stop drinking abruptly or not?)
▶ Work through a range of alternative coping strategies, including the identification of cues that might help distract the patient

⟶ ⟨?⟩ ⟶ Set a quit date?

Phase 5 – Arrange

▶ Be prepared to refer or organise admission to a specialist or appropriate unit if the patient:
  ☐ is in severe withdrawal, including delirium tremens
  ☐ is experiencing unstable social circumstances
  ☐ is likely to develop serious withdrawal due to a severe degree of dependence or a previous episode of severe withdrawal, including delirium tremens
  ☐ is severely dependent
  ☐ has a severe co-morbid physical illness
  ☐ has co-morbid mental illness, including suicidal ideation
  ☐ is using multiple substances
  ☐ has a history of frequent relapse

⟶ ⟨?⟩ ⟶ Need for specialist input?

210

Source: Crome I, Bloor R. Older substance misusers *still* deserve better treatment interventions: an update (part 3) *Reviews in Clinical Gerontology* 2006; **16(1)**: 45–7, reproduced with permission.

Figure 14.2 ○ **Suggested outline for schedule of issues to be covered in assessment**

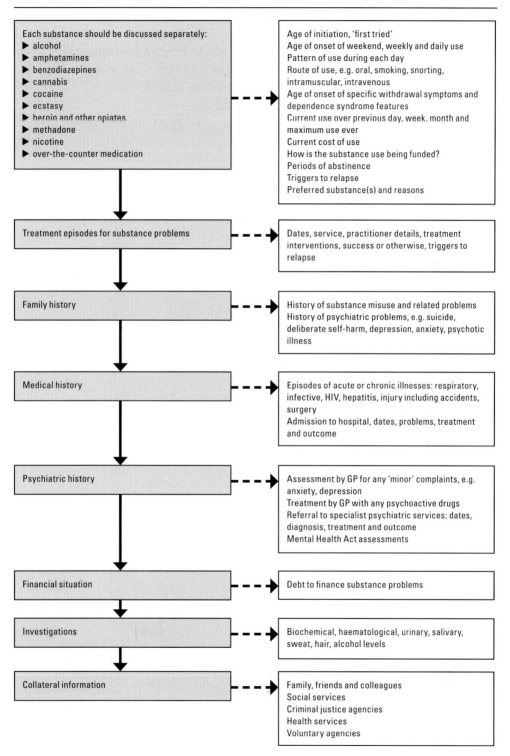

Each substance should be discussed separately:
▶ alcohol
▶ amphetamines
▶ benzodiazepines
▶ cannabis
▶ cocaine
▶ ecstasy
▶ heroin and other opiates
▶ methadone
▶ nicotine
▶ over-the-counter medication

Age of initiation, 'first tried'
Age of onset of weekend, weekly and daily use
Pattern of use during each day
Route of use, e.g. oral, smoking, snorting, intramuscular, intravenous
Age of onset of specific withdrawal symptoms and dependence syndrome features
Current use over previous day, week, month and maximum use ever
Current cost of use
How is the substance use being funded?
Periods of abstinence
Triggers to relapse
Preferred substance(s) and reasons

Treatment episodes for substance problems

Dates, service, practitioner details, treatment interventions, success or otherwise, triggers to relapse

Family history

History of substance misuse and related problems
History of psychiatric problems, e.g. suicide, deliberate self-harm, depression, anxiety, psychotic illness

Medical history

Episodes of acute or chronic illnesses: respiratory, infective, HIV, hepatitis, injury including accidents, surgery
Admission to hospital, dates, problems, treatment and outcome

Psychiatric history

Assessment by GP for any 'minor' complaints, e.g. anxiety, depression
Treatment by GP with any psychoactive drugs
Referral to specialist psychiatric services: dates, diagnosis, treatment and outcome
Mental Health Act assessments

Financial situation

Debt to finance substance problems

Investigations

Biochemical, haematological, urinary, salivary, sweat, hair, alcohol levels

Collateral information

Family, friends and colleagues
Social services
Criminal justice agencies
Health services
Voluntary agencies

211

Source: Crome I, Bloor R. Older substance misusers *still* deserve better treatment interventions: an update (part 3) *Reviews in Clinical Gerontology* 2006; **16(1)**: 45–7, reproduced with permission.

Useful websites

▷ Department of Health, **www.dh.gov.uk/en/Home**.
▷ National Institute for Health and Clinical Excellence, **www.nice.org.uk/**.
▷ National Institute on Drug Abuse (USA), **www.nida.nih.gov/**.
▷ National Treatment Agency for Substance Misuse, **www.nta.nhs.uk/**.
▷ Royal College of Psychiatrists, **www.rcpsych.ac.uk/**.
▷ Scottish Government, **www.scotland.gov.uk/Home**.
▷ Substance Abuse and Mental Health Services Administration (USA), **www.samhsa.gov/**.
▷ Youth Health Talk, **www.youthtalkonline.com/**.

Useful telephone numbers

▷ Al-Anon Family Groups • 0207 928 7377.
▷ Alcohol Concern • 0207 928 7377.
▷ Drinkline • 0800 917 8282.
▷ Families Anonymous • 0207 498 4680.
▷ FRANK • 0800 77 66 00.

References

1 • European Monitoring Centre for Drugs and Drug Addiction. *Drug Use and Related Problems among Very Young People (under 15 Years Old)* Luxembourg: EMCDDA, 2007.

2 • Department for Children, Schools and Families, Home Office, Department of Health. *Youth Alcohol Action Plan* London: The Stationery Office, 2008.

3 • Advisory Council on the Misuse of Drugs. *Pathways to Problems: hazardous use of tobacco, alcohol and other drugs by young people in the UK and its implications for policy* London: Advisory Council on the Misuse of Drugs, 2006.

4 • HM Government. *Drugs: protecting families and communities: the 2008 drug strategy* London: HM Government, 2008, http://drugs.homeoffice.gov.uk/publication-search/drug-strategy/drug-strategy-2008 [accessed August 2009].

5 • Academy of Medical Sciences. *Brain Science, Addiction and Drugs* London: Academy of Medical Sciences, 2008.

6 • HM Government. *Safe. Sensible. Social: the next steps in the National Alcohol Strategy* London: DoH Publications, 2007, www.dh.gov.uk/en/Publicationsandstatistics/Publications/PublicationsPolicyandGuidance/DH_075218 [accessed August 2009].

7 • Nicholas S, Kershaw C, Walker A (eds). *Crime in England and Wales 2006/7* London: Home Office, 2007, www.homeoffice.gov.uk/rds/pdfs07/hosb1107.pdf [accessed August 2009].

8 • Hibell B, Andersson B, Bjarnason T, *et al. The ESPAD Report 2003: alcohol and other drug use among students in 35 European countries* Stockholm: Swedish Council for Alcohol and Other Drugs, 2004.

9 • Cabinet Office. *Alcohol Harm Reduction Strategy for England* London: Cabinet Office, 2004.

10 • Office for National Statistics, Department of Health. *Statistics on Alcohol: England 2004* London: ONS and DoH, 2004.

11 • Office for National Statistics. *General Household Survey 2003* Cardiff: ONS, 2003.

12 • Office for National Statistics. *Smoking Habits in Great Britain* Cardiff: ONS, 2008, www.statistics.gov.uk/cci/nugget.asp?id=313 [accessed August 2009].

13 • Roe S, Man L. *Drug Misuse Declared: findings from the 2005/6 British Crime Survey: England and Wales* London: Home Office, 2006.

14 • Roe S. *Drug Misuse Declared: findings from the 2004/2005 British Crime Survey: England and Wales* London: Home Office, 2005.

15 • Crome I, Ghodse H, Gilvarry E, *et al.* (eds). *Young People and Substance Misuse* London: Gaskell, 2004.

16 • World Health Organization. *International Classification of Diseases 10 (ICD-10)* Geneva: WHO, 1992.

17 • Lingford-Hughes A R, Welch S, Nutt D J. Evidence-based guidelines for the pharmacological management of substance misuse, addiction and comorbidity: recommendations from the British Association for Psychopharmacology *Journal of Psychopharmacology* 2004; **18**: 293–335.

18 • Department of Health, Department of Health, Social Services and Public Safety, Welsh Assembly Government, Scottish Government. *Drug Misuse and Dependence: guidelines on clinical management 2007* London: DoH, 2007.

19 • Crome I B, Christian J, Green C. The development of a unique adolescent community drug service: education, prevention and policy implications *Drugs: education, prevention and policy* 2000; **7**: 87–108.

20 • McIntosh J, MacAskills S, Eadie D, *et al. Evaluation and Description of Drug Projects Working with Young People and Families Funded by Lloyds TSB Foundation Partnership Drugs Initiative* Edinburgh: Scottish Executive, 2006.

21 • McCambridge J, Strang J. The efficacy of single-session motivational interviewing in reducing drug consumption and perceptions of drug-related risk and harm among young people: results from a multi-site cluster randomized trial *Addiction* 2004; **99**: 39–52.

22 • Hammersley R, Reid M, Oliver A., *et al. The National Evaluation of the Youth Justice Board's Drug and Alcohol Projects* London: Youth Justice Board, 2004.

23 • National Institute for Health and Clinical Excellence. *Methadone and Buprenorphine for the Management of Opioid Dependence* (NICE technology appraisal guidance 114) London: NICE, 2007.

24 • National Institute for Health and Clinical Excellence. *Naltrexone for the Management of Opioid Dependence* (NICE technology appraisal guidance 115) London: NICE, 2007.

25 • National Institute for Health and Clinical Excellence. *Clinical Guideline 51, Drug Misuse: psychosocial interventions* London: NICE, 2007, www.nice.org.uk/nicemedia/pdf/ CG051NICEguideline2.pdf [accessed August 2009].

26 • National Institute for Health and Clinical Excellence. *Clinical Guideline 52, Drug Misuse: opioid detoxification* London: NICE, 2007, www.nice.org.uk/nicemedia/pdf/DrugMisuseOpioidDetoxFullGuidelinePublishedVersion.pdf [accessed August 2009].

27 • Brown S A, D'Amico E J, McCarthy D M, *et al*. Four-year outcomes from adolescent alcohol and drug treatment *Journal of Studies on Alcohol* 2001; **62**: 381–8.

28 • Chung T, Maisto S A, Cornelius J R, *et al*. Adolescents' drug and alcohol use trajectories in the year following treatment *Journal of Studies on Alcohol* 2004; **65**: 105–14.

29 • Williams R J, Chang S Y. A comprehensive and comparative review of adolescent substance abuse treatment outcome *Clinical Psychology: science and practice* 2000; **7**: 138–66.

30 • Hser Y-I, Grella C E, Hubbard R L, *et al*. An evaluation of drug treatments for adolescents in 4 US cities *Archives of General Psychiatry* 2001; **58**: 689–95.

31 • New Zealand Health Technology Assessment. *Adolescent Therapeutic Day Programmes and Community-Based Programmes for Serious Mental Illness and Serious Drug and Alcohol Problems: a critical appraisal of the literature* Christchurch: Department of Public Health and General Practice, Christchurch School of Medicine, 1998, http://nzhta.chmeds.ac.nz/publications/dayprog.pdf [accessed August 2008].

32 • Liddle H A, Dakof G A, Turner R M, *et al*. Treating adolescent drug abuse: a randomized trial comparing multidimensional family therapy and cognitive behaviour therapy *Addiction* 2008; **103**: 1660–70.

33 • Henggeler S W, Halliday-Boykins C A, Cunningham P B, *et al*. Juvenile drug court: enhancing outcomes by integrating evidence-based treatments *Journal of Consulting and Clinical Psychology* 2006; **74**: 42–54.

34 • Waldron H B, Kaminer Y. On the learning curve: the emerging evidence supporting cognitive-behavioral therapies for adolescent substance abuse *Addiction* 2004; **99**: 93–105.

35 • Dennis M, Godley S H, Diamond G, *et al*. The Cannabis Youth Treatment (CYT) study: main findings from two randomized trials *Journal of Substance Abuse Treatment* 2004; **27**: 197–213.

36 • Tait R J, Hulse G K. A systematic review of the effectiveness of brief interventions with substance using adolescents by type of drug *Drug and Alcohol Review* 2003; **22**: 337–46.

37 • Mirza K A H, McArdle P, Crome I B, *et al*. (eds). *The Role of CAMHS and Addiction Psychiatry in Adolescent Substance Misuse Services* London: National Treatment Agency for Substance Misuse, 2008.

38 • National Treatment Agency for Substance Misuse. *Young People's Substance Misuse Treatment Services: essential elements* London: National Treatment Agency for Substance Misuse, 2005.

39 • Royal College of Psychiatrists and Royal College of General Practitioners' Joint Substance Misuse Working Group. *Roles and Responsibilities of Doctors in the Provision of Treatment for Drug and Alcohol Misusers* (Council Report CR131) London: RCPsych, 2005.

Index